# *Strong as Death…*

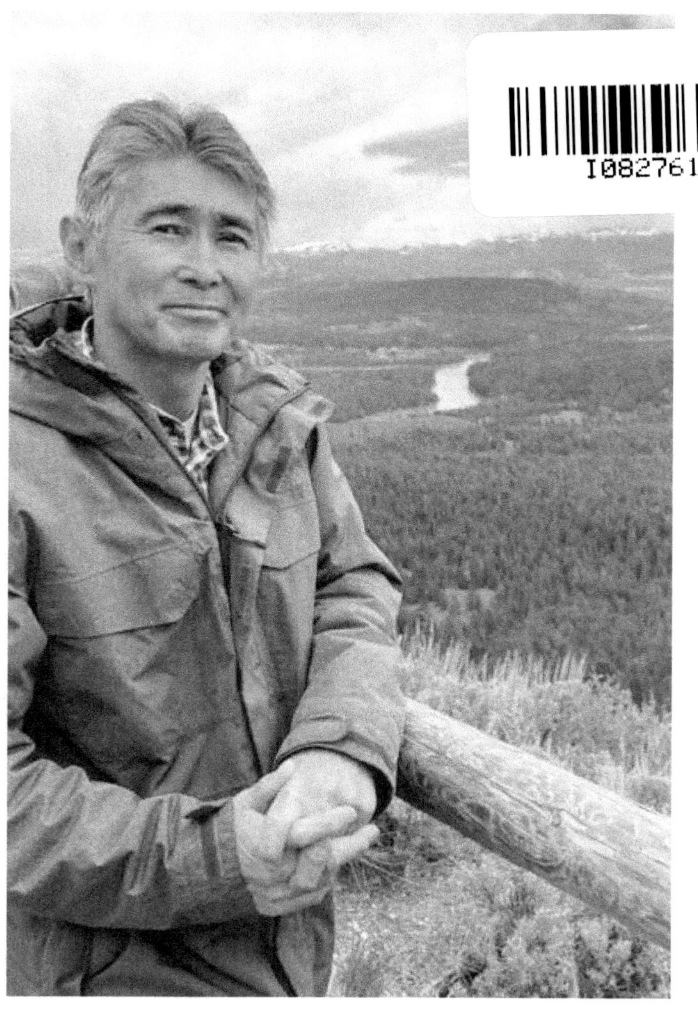



Michael Yanuck MD PhD

**ISBN: 978-1-946600-47-9**

## DEDICATION

In memory of Sam Morishima,
Friend and mentor,
July 13, 1953 – August 14, 2025

*Yea Strong as Death is Love…*
*~Song of Solomon 8:6*

*Hi everyone,*

*My best friend and confidante, Sam, is having significant pain and difficulties breathing. So, on Sunday, May 11, 2025 (Mother's Day), I insisted he let me take him to Stanford University to be evaluated at their Emergency Room (ER). Really, I mostly wanted the ER visit to facilitate a Pulmonary referral, because second opinions from Stanford had been exceedingly helpful to members for my family, like my father for his brain tumor, and mother-in-law for her heart condition. As it happened, though, Sam's difficulties breathing were so severe that he was admitted to the hospital immediately, and following several tests, he was told his lung condition was so advanced that there was nothing they could do.*

*As you know from my earlier writings, Sam has been at the heart of my most important breakthroughs in Qi Gong, and it's hard for me to imagine life without him.*

*It's nighttime now, and I plan to flood the airwaves with stories of the intense moments I've been living through - or, more appropriately, Sam's been living through.*

*I'll begin where I left off, with Sam advising me to go to Yale, and then, move to the present. Here we go…*

# CHAPTER ONE

As plans neared for me to leave for the fellowship at Yale, I confided to Sam (as usual) about hurdles involved in the process.

Although in a recent conversation with Ellen (who oversaw the Yale VA program), she assured me that, in spite of the government cuts, her program was up and running; however, she didn't have a mentor for me yet. She thought that she could find one (because she said she'd always been successful at that in the past), but I wasn't sure.

Only a year ago, I'd let go of the fellowship because of obstacles to teaching my Qi Gong approach there. At the time, my wife, April, was argued that if Yale was getting in the way of that, then I might as well stay in northern California, where I was permitted to train folks in my approach.

"April is right about that," Sam commented.

Yes, but since the successful Innovation Accelerator Qi Gong project (in which Veterans had been helped with my Qi Gong approach for TBI, neurologic deficits, chronic pain, opioid dependence and long COVID), the Northern California VA hadn't given me any dedicated time to continue my Qi Gong efforts, whereas Ellen was promising she'd make my Qi Gong activities 80% of what I did at Yale.

Sam asked how Ellen "rated" compared to other folks I'd worked with? I responded that, in my gut, I believed Ellen was just the kind of person I needed to give me "wings to fly."

"You're definitely on the right course," Sam said. "The reason why you stayed here last year was to finish the [UC Davis Long COVID-Qi Gong] study. Remember, this study was vital, and it turned out better than you expected. It was worth staying here. For you to have walked out at the beginning of that study would have been the biggest mistake of your life.

"So, there you are: There was a good reason you stayed. The reason you stayed here was to get that study done. And that justified everything.

"And Ellen recognized that, because now your study is her study. If that study had turned out negative, you probably would've gone back to being depressed and saying, 'What am I doing?' You would've probably changed your course. You'd be focused on just doing your job."

But I didn't agree; I felt if I'd made a difference in the lives of one or two of the study participants, it would have been enough for me.

"No, not for what you're trying to do," Sam declared. "Not for what you're trying to do, Mike. One or two is a fluke. It's placebo. It's whatever. But what you did was outstanding. And it shows the positive effect of this - The potential."

"Ellen is not stupid," he concluded. "She recognizes that. So, therefore – BOOM - that's why she needs you. And that's why you need her…"

# CHAPTER TWO

I told Sam that Ellen had asked the question of whether, within my Qi Gong work, I thought there was a spiritual element? I tried to defer, saying it was mostly about working at the level of the energetic circulation, which I consider the potential last and final frontier of human physiology that we have yet to be able to measure.

I did, however, ask her why she asked the question? She said it was because there was a Yale-Trinity school connection, and she was wondering about avenues for making connections?

"I think you need to make those connections," Sam responded. "But I think you need to be focused. To me, there are three aspects of Qi Gong: There's the health aspect; there's the spiritual or religious aspect; and then, there is the martial arts aspect. You're not concerned with the martial arts, unless the martial arts can contribute to health. The spirituality aspect - You should not worry about that either, unless there are some aspects of that have a health component. For you, the key thing is the health aspect. I mean, you should be able to dissociate the martial arts and the spiritual or religious aspects from the health aspects."

True, though even back when I was working on the cancer vaccine, I'd had thought about the "hereafter"; namely, when the research was taking off, so that there was the prospect of finding a vaccine that would significantly curtail the ravages of cancer, it crossed my mind, "OK, we might be able to cure cancer. But what then? How are we going to cure death?"

And then, my leg was injured, and I experienced chronic pain, and this led me to Qi Gong and the life-changing experience that led me to believe that life was about a spirit entity learning the lessons of the universe on the physical plane; and in that way, Qi Gong answered an existential question that had been plaguing me, and it took that weight off of me, so that I was better able to live my life with less fear of death. Hence, long story short, it did seem to me that Qi Gong offered an important spiritual element.

"Yes," Sam replied. "Like I said, those things, if they have the capability of enhancing health are important. But otherwise, no."

"There are people who are not going to be in Qi Gong for the spirituality," he continued, "and definitely not for the martial arts aspects of it. But yet need it. And why? It's because it contributes to health. If the other things can contribute to health for an individual, let them. But those are individual things.

"Somebody who loves physical exercise will use the martial arts aspect of Qi Gong to help enhance their health and make them jump higher, and chin up better, or whatever. Help them get psychological self-confidence to beat someone else. Fine. But it's not going to do any good for their health if the health aspect isn't there. The health aspect has to be there.

"It's just like everybody says: When you get older, the only thing that people think about is their health. Then, they say, 'Health is everything', and everything else follows. They say, 'I need my health, so I can go to church', and 'I need my health so that I can spiritually help people', and 'I need my health, so that I can physically defend myself against violent attackers.' Health is number one. That's where your concentration and focus should be. If you can add those other things in, then great, as long as you have the health aspect. You're going there to improve people's health..."

# CHAPTER THREE

"I think the moment that you get over there, you're going to be so immersed in your work that you won't be able to think about very much anything else," Sam declared. "At least for the first two or three years."

Yes, that was the duration of the fellowship.

"Good thing that you're still young," he added.

I wasn't young. Indeed, most people (including my wife) thought I was crazy to enter a research fellowship at my age and stage of life, being just a few years from retirement. But when I'd let go of the fellowship a year ago, I'd rather entered something of a depression; and, yes, winding up homeless, because our landlord insisted we leave even when I didn't have the fellowship to go to could have been part of it; but it wasn't until Ellen reached back to me and asked if I was still interested in the fellowship that I got out from under that dark cloud.

"I think people are starting to realize your value," Sam responded. "And well-deserved, because you've worked so hard. You haven't given up. Your tenacity to move on with this has been extraordinary. I don't think they're going to find anybody like you. Or they may, but it's going to be a really rare find - someone with your set of experiences and everything that you've done.

"I think Ellen realizes that, and she has to really try hard to rope you in. Because her best chances of succeeding in her lifetime is dependent on people like you.

"The problem is the other people you need... Well, you're going to have to find them. You're going to have to develop a team of doctors of BioEnerQi."

I said I regarded that as something to look forward to.

"Exciting times!" he declared. "I just hope you're going to be well compensated for it. Maybe not right now, but eventually."

I told Sam that the possibility of going to God being able to say I did my best to do what He/She put me in the world for was compensation enough, and as I did, a shiver ran down my spine.

"You have to do better than best," Sam insisted. "You're going to have to make a difference."

Did I? I responded. Even my formerly harsh and overbearing father was inclined to tell me, "The best you can do is the best you can do."

"Well, yeah, that's what you have to do," he responded. "But in the end, you gotta make a difference… And I think you will. And I think Yale will get you there faster..."

# CHAPTER FOUR

Sam asserted that might have been a blessing in disguise that our previous landlord kicked us out of our former rental by the river.

"Because now it will be an easier move for you, since all your belongings are in storage," he asserted. "It's better to take things in steps."

"It's amazing," he added. "Some people would always say that there's a reason for what's happening. 'God has a purpose. God has a plan.' But I don't believe in that. I think things happen, and we've got to make the best of it. So, might as well make the best of this situation that you have."

Then, Sam commented this was the first time I'd shared that the Yale fellowship was back on.

"That's so exciting," he said, spiritedly. "So exciting."

What a friend, I thought. He's not worried about what that means for him - losing me to a move to a different state on the other side of the country - He just wants what's best for me. What a friend...

# CHAPTER FIVE

I shared my concerns about a Yale official, who I'll refer to as Dr. A., who raised the issues that led me to abort my plans to go to the Yale VA last year. Reconnecting with her this year, she listened to my International Congress to presentation with a Cheshire cat smile, and, in the end, pounced, telling me that she still didn't consider what I did external Qi Gong, because it was influenced by my Bioenergy background.

"It sounds like you don't feel she's very supportive," Sam deduced. "But she's not actively against you. She's just trying to limit you and see what you come up with. The feeling I get is that she wants to see what outcomes you have. And then, she'll make her judgment. But right now, she's kind of leery and wants to be careful where you're concerned.

"But I think you'll prove to her that this really works, and there's a method to this, and once we fine tune this method, you'll discover something practical."

Still, it made nervous, and I harbored a lot of hard feelings for her having waited to the last minute to sink my project a year ago.

"Mike, I believe that she's not against you," Sam reiterated. "She's just being very cautious, and she does have some concerns that your approach needs to be validated? And she's wondering if you're willing to go through that validation process and make modifications if you're Qi Gong approach is significantly different from other people's external Qi Gog approaches? Or if you're so headstrong that you want to do it a certain way that you have right now and not really change as things happen to make it better? This is the way that I would look at it if someone came up to me, and I was running the program: I would wonder if they were willing to modify their approach?"

I wasn't particularly willing to modify my practice. I'd been perfecting it for 30 years and believed it was the best external Qi Gong approach.

"The thing is," Sam asserted, "I think everything is too early to make conclusions about anything. I hope DR. A. will give you the freedom to start working and see what the results show.

"I mean, everything seems to be so embryonic that no one knows what this embryo is going to turn out to be when it grows up? Or if it survives? I think she's putting up a lot of resistance to you, but that resistance will fade as she gets to know you and starts seeing your work."

Sam asked if they had any definition for bioenergy?

I laughed, because aside from what I'd written about my training and experiences with bioenergy under Dr. Rind, there was no documentation of it at all.

For years, I'd asked Dr. Rind to write a letter of reference for me; however, in spite of these requests, he'd never written a word to substantiate any claims that he'd trained me in bioenergy 30 years ago. Hence, I had no certificates in bioenergy. Nothing. For all anyone really knew, I'd made it all up.

"Then, at this point, I would drop bioenergy, and say, 'I'm just practicing Qi Gong'," he advised. "You can go on and say, 'I do have a belief that there may be another component to this, which is bioenergy, but we haven't defined it yet, and the main focus is Qi Gong, and we'll see what comes out of it?'

"It's like it was when people first worked with atomic particles: They didn't know about photons and neutrons and electrons and quarks, until they started working with it. So, before it was like, 'There's the atom', and then they started discovering other particles."

"So, bioenergy isn't defined yet," he concluded. "And my question is, what is the reason that they want you over there?"

Ellen wants to expand the Complementary and Integrative Medicine approaches available to help people with problems of addiction, and that included advancing my work in Qi Gong. She wants me to study this approach and see if it helps people.

"Right," he said. "So, I don't know how this other woman DR. A. can oppose you if you're bringing this method that works? It seems to me that later, if they find that there's a component to bioenergy, and they define what bioenergy is - or you define it - then they can take that into account."

**"I mean, to be honest with you, I don't know what she's arguing about, really?" he asked. "Except for her view of what you are, it has nothing to do with what you're really trying to work on?"**

**Whatever it was, she was an obstacle, and I was afraid of that.**

**"Yeah, but you have to deal with her," he declared. "You're going to be living in the same house with her. But the question is, Are you guys going to be able to get along enough that you can move about and do the things that you need to do?"**

**"Anyway, take my words with a grain of salt," he added. "I'm glad to hear you tell me that Dr. A. isn't fully against you, but has some reservations. I think those reservations are good things. Because if you could overcome her reservations… Well, I'm going to tell you, my best customers when I was in the medical field and was trying to expand our products into the laboratories, were the ones who gave me the hardest time at the beginning to all of our sales reps, so that people hated them.**

**"And so, those people got sent to me, since I was the marketing director. And I worked with them. And once I overcame their objections, and they incorporated our system into their laboratories, they became my strongest allies. And they became my opinion leaders and gave me my strongest testimonials."**

**"So, Dr. A. will turn into that," he concluded. "If you do everything right, she won't be able to help becoming your strongest ally..."**

# CHAPTER SIX

Sam commented about the larger issue that I'd be facing at Yale.

"There's a lot of medical people who won't believe you," he said. "I'm going to tell you, they're won't. I'm just going to make that statement that there's going to be a certain percentage of those people who really will not.

"And it comes in different types of people: First, there are people who believe what they think and feel is the correct thing, even when it's not.

"Then, there are the people who say, 'Yeah, I feel it', but they really don't and are just saying that to get through it. Like the person who's taking Chemistry as part of their pre-med requirements: That person doesn't really care if he knows that shit; he just cares that he passes it, and the teacher gives him a passing grade. There's a lot of those people. So, they pass it. And so, you assume they know chemistry. Because why? They got a passing grade. But they barely passed the test. But that they got the passing grade is all that matters. Study just enough. They don't really understand it, but enough to answer the true or false questions, and a few diagrams, etc. There are people like that. And you're going to find them in every discipline.

"Then, there's also people who just want to make money. They think, 'This is a great way to make money, and I'll get to know people, too.'

"And it's that way with any discipline. That's why you have great doctors and you have mediocre ones. You try to minimize that by medical schools requiring them to pass a certain level of capability and knowledge, so that they can say, 'Yeah, OK, they're not the greatest, or the sharpest tool in the shed, but they are now an instrument that can perform most of their chores and maybe that's good enough?'

"So, Mike, it's going to be your responsibility, since you're working on all of this, to develop a rigorous checks and balances of the process, so that when people are performing it, they're doing it properly. And then you have to put guard rails up, so that it's not susceptible to quackery. You have to set up certain tasks to have them perform consistently, through repetitive work, so that it doesn't just work on one patient. And that's why you're doing clinical research - so that you can work on many different people with different conditions.

"And then, you need a person who actually checks your work and serve as your mentor in your fellowship. And they all need to understand the process and what they're doing and be able to explain why the process works and how the process works.

"There's many things that have to be done. And just saying, 'Yeah, you're doing it right. I certify you', is not a way to ensure that your methodology will be accepted out in the real world and be used appropriately. If anything, there's a chance for failure of the whole system that way. And your system actually works and doesn't deserve any negative associations that would crush or bury it.

"I want you to succeed, because as I know you – You keep reinforcing positive indications that this is a viable medical process. I don't see anything that you've done that has caused me to say, 'Whoa, this is really bad stuff and shouldn't be used.' Every time you work with me, and the things you've done with other people - Kino and with the study and others - you've just been producing positive results."

"So," he concluded, "I'd just hate to see it get destroyed..."

# CHAPTER SEVEN

I had to get on the road, as I had plans to visit my father, who was having worsening problems of dementia. Before ending the call, Sam said the next time I saw him, he wanted to take me to his favorite Chinese dumpling restaurant.

It struck me that whereas I used to see Sam daily, now I hadn't seen Sam in over a year.

Also, this had significance for me, because among the last things I did with my first Qi Gong mentor, Wah Lee (who had recently passed away), was let him take April and me to his favorite Chinese dumpling restaurant in Chinatown, DC.

"I don't know if I should be treated like a mentor," Sam said. "Just take what I say with a grain of salt."

"I have no intention of mentoring you," he added, "nor any intention of making you any better or smarter. I'm just giving you my opinion.

"And coming back to the dumplings, I just thought that before you left Sacramento, I should at least have you go to this place and try out something that I think is pretty darn good."

"So, whenever you're in the neighborhood," he concluded, "look me up?..."

# CHAPTER EIGHT

While visiting with my father, I got concerned for my dad and others I'd be leaving to take the Yale position.

Confiding to Sam, he responded this way:

"Getting lost and stuck in the past is easy to do," he began. "It requires energy to move out of that. I mean, it's good to enjoy that and have that, but not to be chained to it. And, so, you have to put in some energy to break the chain and move forward. Because being in the present is important – and also the future. More important than being in the past.

"Probably most important is how do you divide your time? Put 15% of your energy in the past. And 70% in the present. And another 15% into the future – because you can't ignore the future, because the future will eventually become the present – and then the past. So, the more you can mold the future, you can have a more predictable present and past.

"I keep on thinking - when I think of you - you have a vision for the future for yourself. And I think you just need to focus and get some more clarity to it, so that when it becomes the present, you can make greater opportunities from it.

"One of the things to get that energy to get out of the past is to find something in the past that you can stand on. It's like Newton Third Law: For every action, there's an equal and opposite reaction. So, therefore, to be able to jump forward or higher, you have to be standing on something."

Yes, I was standing on his belief in me. I was standing on his desire to see me succeed in all of my dreams. He gifted me the funding for the University of California-Davis Long COVID-Qi Gong study, which was found to impart statistically significant

**improvements to long COVID sufferers for problems of fatigue, pain, activity tolerance, shortness of breath, anxiety and depression. I could stand on that and take that into the future - By honoring his gift to me when it came to these things.**

**"So, I would say, go into the past to get something that you can stand on," Sam continued. "So that once you could stand on something, you could deal with the present in a more stable manner, and that will also allow you to leap off a bit into the future. So that the purpose of your past is to go back and get something that you had stored away that you can use. Because you kept it there for future use. And so your past has a value for your present and for your future, and that's how the relationship with the past is.**

**"Or else the past has all kinds of stuff, and you can be a hoarder who never finds anything that you specifically want in an efficient and timely manner – So that you can go back and get something of value, and keep your past organized, so that you can find things quicker and better that you need.**

**"Because that's what memories are for. And that's what dreams are for. To help you organize the value of your past, so that you can deal with the present and future in a more constructive, productive and efficient manner.**

**"And it brings joy! Because you didn't lose the past. In fact, you are incorporating it, so that it has a greater part and value to you for the present and future. And so it helps shape who you are. And, therefore the past creates who you are today."**

**"Again, when I think of you, I think you have such a bright future," he asserted. "Very few people have futures they can actually use. It's like a rope: Somebody dropped a rope for you, and that's the future. And that rope allows you to climb higher. You just need to know how to climb up the rope. That's all.**

**"Again, very few people have a rope to the future that is dropped down for them to use to go higher. Most people find that they have no future."**

**I thought of my father and his dementia and persistent cognitive decline. The night before, he kept on talking about wanting to fly a plane again, and all the joy that gave him in the past, but he doesn't have the faculties to engage in that activity anymore – ever…**

**"They have no rope," Sam continued. "And then there are some people who use that rope to hang themselves, because they don't take opportunities with the rope, or because they don't use it properly. So, you have to decide how you're going to use that rope."**

**I think I'll climb it to a brighter place, I thought.**

**"Nothing is 100%," Sam concluded. "And a lot of it is dependent on what you do with it..."**

# CHAPTER NINE

There have been rumblings coming out of Yale that my position was not certain. In spite of this, I was still working towards the position, feeling if the worst happens and it all falls apart, maybe somewhere down the line, people will appreciate that I gave it a try.

"Oh, I'm glad you're thinking this way," Sam commented. "Because that's exactly what you need to do. I just didn't want you to be discouraged. Because I think the times are definitely not in your favor."

"I'm not saying that they're against you," he added. "I just think they're not a favorable environment, that's all."

Sam compared my difficulties with those created for him by the highway construction near his house.

"It's like one more thing that I have to take into consideration for the rest of my life," he said. "And I can't work around it."

"These times right now are really weird, and I just can't understand how we've allowed one person to have all this power and causing this ripple effect? It's sort of like a bolder was tossed into this nice, still, calm lake, and this ripple goes from the epicenter goes to every shore."

"So, they're not making a very smooth road for you," he said, returning to the situation at Yale. "That's all I'm saying. So be careful in these times. Don't give up. You just need to walk this path in a very, very wise manner and look out for all the obstacles in your way."

Then, he described his worsening respiratory condition.

"Every breath is work for me now," he concluded. "It's become my centerpiece. And everything else is secondary to it..."

# CHAPTER TEN

Sam talked about wanting to share his knowledge with others but feeling stymied.

He had been caring for his grandson at the time, and I commented that, at some point, perhaps he could share his interests with him, perhaps starting with his knowledge of the Rubik's cube?

Sam responded that his grandson had little interest in that right now.

"I could show him how to move the blocks in a very simplistic way," he said. "When he was first doing it, he couldn't change the blocks. But now he can, because I give it to him every time I see him, and now he's able to move a layer. But moving a layer and solving the puzzle are two different things and a freaking long way apart. But at least I gave him a little bit of a head start."

Sam described working with his grandson on balance.

"It was interesting," he began. "He was at a party, and all the parents were amazed at him, because all the kids were trying to walk the I-beam, and he walks it very relaxed with his feet, one in front of the other, and just walks across, whereas the other kids couldn't do it."

"So that gives him a little head start to take up skiing at a later age," he concluded. "I may not be there, but at least I gave him something."

I thought his grandson was very lucky.

"It's not the same as sharing with someone who wants to learn something," he added. "Because, in this case, you want to share it with them so much, but you can't. You can only show them a teeny tiny fraction of it."

**Just then, I heard his grandson come back to the room, and Sam excused himself, so he could get back to attending him...**

## CHAPTER ELEVEN

I confided that I was becoming concerned that by playing it safe and entering the Yale fellowship in October with the new fiscal year, I might miss out on it altogether.

"I think even if I could do the fellowship for just one day, I want that one day," I said, "rather than risk that fellowship going away at the beginning of the next fiscal year and not having had the opportunity to participate in it at all."

"Look," he responded, "everything's up in the air, and it can get worse, and it can get better. You just got to take what you feel excited about and do what you need to do and deal with the consequences as things come up.

"I don't think you're really secure anywhere. If you're looking for a security, then you should try to look for something that's as secure as possible. But realizing that nothing is really secure... Well, even where there seems to be a degree of security, that degree might be fickle, because things that don't seem secure might be, and things that seem not to be secure, may be a lot more secure than you think.

"So, it's one of those things where you try to use your logic and judgment as well as possible. But you've got to also take risks and do things that you want to get done in your life.

"So, it's a risky time. Either way you can fall into a trap. And you can become very successful and make the right judgments on the path of your life, as well. Both are possible. You just have to use the combination of logic and a little bit of emotion and passion where you want. It's a very complicated formula, and the variables that you put weight on are really dependent on you.

"So, it sounds like you're saying you might want to delay your satisfaction for the sake of security. And I tell you, we're at a

**crossroads right now. So, you got to determine what things are most important to you. But at least you have options. You're a lucky guy. Most people don't, and they can't deviate from the path that they're on.**

**"So, are you going to say, 'I'm lucky I have options, but I don't need to take those options', or, 'I have these options, and I may take one of those options', or, 'I will take one of those options.' You've got a lot of reflecting to do, Mike.**

**"Because it seems like things keeps on going up and down on you. But with all of this up and down, I think it's taking you closer to an answer…"**

# CHAPTER TWELVE

I told Sam that trips to my father's were about giving my stepmother a reprieve, being that my father wouldn't accept assistance from others, insisting, "I don't need a babysitter", but he does!

"I know that he thinks he can do it, but that's an illusion," Sam responded. "It makes him feel good, but he's not really able to do it. He can do it to an extent, but he can't do it completely. So, it's an illusion. And sometimes we like to live in the illusion. So, what makes your dad happy is his illusion."

Yes. Indeed, I still kicking myself about an evening that my stepmother and I had a tense encounter, and my father overheard me saying he didn't have the cognitive ability to function independently.

*"Don't treat him like he should be able to remember things," I'd told her. "He can't."*

*"Why can't I remember things?" my father then asked.*

*I spoke in truisms in the unsparing way he'd spoke to me all my life, saying it was because he had a problem with the wiring and neural circuitry in his brain, such that the part of the brain that took information from the present and transferred into memory storage.*

*"Well, why isn't that happening?" he asked.*

*I don't know Dad, I responded. I can only imagine that the neural wiring there got shorted-out somehow.*

*"Damaged," he responded, matter-of-factly. "Just no longer working..."*

"And how did your dad take that?" Sam asked.

**He seemed to accept it as information, I responded. Statement of fact. But I was still upset at myself for having said something hurtful to him.**

**"Well, I doubt that he'll remember that conversation," Sam responded.**

**Probably not. And maybe I shouldn't feel so bad about this anyway, because it is rather important information after all. Because the state of denial that he was in was keeping him from getting appropriate help. Help they could potentially make his life more pleasant.**

**But I don't want him to be sad. I don't want to bring him down. I want him to have pleasant experiences in this time. Not sad ones.**

**In the end, it seemed I did want him to be in a place of pleasant illusions.**

**"My answer to that is," Sam began, "you know he needs help, and it's not just him, but it's also your stepmother. It would make life easier for her, too. And it's just a matter of time that you're going to get hospice care. Sometimes you have to bite the bullet now, rather than wait till later. So that you can get the care now, and feel better now, instead of waiting for some accident, so that it becomes an emergency."**

**"As they say," he concluded, "'A little bit of preventive medicine can eliminate a lot of unnecessary suffering'."**

**I thought about those times that my father fell from the roof, and the surgeries he required because of that. Those surgeries might have contributed to his dementia, and if he just would have spent a little bit of money to hire someone to do that work on the roof, those injuries wouldn't have happened.**

**In any event, getting ahead of something was the smart thing to do, rather than waiting for some catastrophe to happen.**

**"I always thought so," Sam responded.**

**He confided about his mother and how it was that she was receiving hospice care.**

**"And we try to get it for her as soon as we can," he said. "And it makes life easier for her. It makes life easier for everybody. Because the nurse comes in and sees her every other week and gives her a bath. And my family gives her a bath, but it's one bath that my sisters and my brother don't have to give her. And that takes some of the stress off of them."**

**"It all depends on how much pain tolerance your stepmother is willing to accept," he declared. "If she's willing to do everything… Well, as you know, the quality of those things will begin to dwindle."**

**Yes, I was concerned about my stepmother and her tolerance for my father's memory difficulties.**

**"Yeah, but that's because she's being overloaded," Sam said...**

# CHAPTER THIRTEEN

Taking a stroll outside, I heard music coming from a home across the street from where we were living in Davis, and I found the voice of the woman singing so extraordinary (like she was making these old songs her own!) that I went walking in that direction. In particular, the singer's voice reminded me of Krissy Hines from the Pretenders, who was my female favorite and whose voice I'd fall asleep to in my adolescence.

The gate to the backyard of the house was open; but as I was about to go inside, I bumped into an older man, who told me the concert was free, but the average age of those inside was about 15 and it was mostly girls.

"That's not good," I responded.

But my desire to offer my praise to the vocalist was was such that it overpowered my better judgment.

At the gate, I was greeted by a young Asian woman who told me that the event was being sponsored by a sorority, and when I expressed my appreciation for the vocalist, she told me her name was Bernadette from a local band called Cowboys after Dark, and she would be happy to introduce me to her.

Bernadette was a sweet, tall, young, dark haired woman of color, which was not what I was expecting (I was expecting a "ballsy blonde"!).

After expressing my appreciation for her singing, I was invited to stay. But felt out of place – though, later, I realized this was mostly stemming from my experiences in Sacramento, where it was my impression that young people didn't want me at venues like this – though this certainly wasn't my feeling there.

"Davis is a college town!" Sam exclaimed. "Right there, you have a certain level of academia, so that all these young people are dealing with professors, who they admire and respect, and know that older people have experience and knowledge, that they listen to.

"So, you have a whole different demographic of people in Davis for one thing, versus Sacramento, where they don't have much respect for older people on average. In fact, they're more rebellious against older people, whereas kids in a college town have a bit more respect for older people. So, I can understand that. It's a generalization, but that's what I find when I walk around Davis."

"Also, in a college town, it's not just the college kids, but also the residents who live there. They're more family oriented."

Yes, I said, and I preferred this over what I'd found in Sacramento.

"I know," Sam said, understandingly. "I know you do. That's why I thought you'd love living in Davis. You asked me about other places in Sacramento to live when you were moving out, and even in my neighborhood? And it would've been nice to have you in my neighborhood, but I was happier when you said you were going to Davis.

"Because here you are thinking of going to Yale. You still have that academic mind. That youthfulness. You need to be more in that environment.

"Sacramento is a little bit more settled. I'm living in Curtis Park, and here you'd be living in a higher academic level. But the people here are settled, and the thinking is more of, I don't want to say retirement, but it's past the point of academic endeavors, and more of just getting into the rat race. And here you are thinking about going to Yale and getting a fellowship…"

## CHAPTER FOURTEEN

"You see," he continued. "I think of people like you in this area as kind of like a knife: when you're studying, you want to have a sharp mind. And so, you need to be cutting things with the knife in an area where you have good sharpening stones. And that's like Davis: There are places where you use your sharp blade, your knife, and there are so many honing stones that allow you to hone your blade and keep it sharp. Whereas in Sacramento, the only thing you have are things that keep dulling your knife, and very little honing stones that are nearby that allow you to sharpen your blade. So, you need to be in an environment that has both capabilities – Allowing you to cut, but also to rejuvenate and hone that blade to keep it sharp, keep it tuned. And that's what the Davis area does.

"So, what you were talking about – the young people - They're sharpening your blade for you. Whereas the people in Sacramento are dulling your blade."

At the very least, it seemed my experiences in Sacramento were leading me to close doors on myself: I didn't want to go out and listen to music; I didn't want to go out dancing; I didn't want to go out doing karaoke. I felt rejected, and I was acting on that rejection.

"In your present position at the VA, it seems they keep acting to make you want to dull your blade - They keep using your knife until it gets dull, and they don't give you the opportunity to hone and sharpen it."

I didn't think Sam was cognizant of those issues or recall that I'd ever confided about feeling like my present boss wasn't utilizing my expertise in homelessness, pain and addiction; instead it felt like he was putting me in a box, confined to my exam room, so that it wasn't at all like my first years, when I was going out into the field and making a difference in the lives of homeless veterans; he wasn't letting me do projects, like the VA Innovation Accelerator project that brought my abilities in Qi Gong to light; he wasn't letting me lead pain and opioid use initiatives; instead, he was just dumping more and more routine patients on me.

"If you want to have a sharp mind and a sharp knife," Sam said, "you're going to have to go to the place where they're going to sharpen it for you. Are you going to get that sharpening at the VA here? Or are you going to get it over there at Yale?"

The answer was obvious. I was nervous, though; I thought I would miss being a big fish in a small pond. I mean, look at how much I'd accomplished here: The VA innovation accelerator project; the UC Davis Long Covid Qi Gong study. Would that happen at Yale? Or was I going to be treated like some guy who came with a bag of tricks and a lot of pseudoscience who no one was interested in? And I was scared about being far away from Sam and the rest of my rooting section.

"Yeah, there are going to be some losses," Sam acknowledged. "But, again, you just have to weigh everything: What are you willing to sacrifice to get other things? Everybody sacrifices something. There's nothing that allows you to maintain everything 100%.

"Look, the way I look at it, to sharpen a good knife, if you want it to be surgically capable, you have to use a finer grit stone to sharpen it. You have to know first how dull your blade is, and then you put the appropriate coarse grit on it to get it to a certain sharpness. Then, you get finer and finer grit. There's something that they call the Arkansas stone, which is a sharpening stone that has such a fine grit that it's sharpen your blade to a razor sharp edge. In Sacramento, there's no Arkansas stones. But you can find that stone most likely at Yale. So, it all depends on how sharp you want to get your blade?

"The thing is, though, most people are comfortable with normal sharpening: They're don't to be doing things to make their knife too sharp – because then they're potentially cutting themselves. But you can't use it as a sushi knife, because it won't cut the fish that thin and cleanly. So, it all depends on how sharp a knife you want to be..."

# CHAPTER FIFTEEN

I asked Sam how he was doing?

"Oh, I'd say I'm pretty dull," he said, continuing on the knife analogy. "Anyway, I'm not actually in the knife business anymore. I'm more in the hammer business."

"It's going to get really bad soon," he declared. "So, you may want to be in a more protective environment, which Yale might provide. Too bad you're not going to Harvard."

I confided to Sam that any time I'd ever been in Massachusetts, it always felt so cold to me (so to make Connecticut feel like the subtropics!) and I didn't think I could tolerate the weather there.

"Yeah, it gets cold," he affirmed, tepidly. "But the thing is, no place is perfect. And the object is not so that you can enjoy your environment; it's to be able to get what you want out of your academic studies - And move on.

"Because life is a continuum. It's just like, when you go to school, you give up a lot of things in life. But a lot of times, for most people, they make it up. They graduate, and then they see the world in a much more open and detailed way because of their education and ability to work at something.

"And the reason that you do work - and you do want to get paid! - is because it will provide for a better life in the future.

"You of all people should know that you've sacrificed a lot to have a better life. If you were someone who said right out of high school, 'I'm going to start enjoying my life, and school is going to be a drag on me', then you would have gone off and traveled and saw the world and not gone to school. And some people are successful doing that. But more people are not. You can be working at some automobile assembly line. Not that you couldn't be happy, but it would be a different kind of happiness."

I told Sam that at this point I did feel like I was working on a factory line.

"Yeah, but it's so much cleaner factory line," he countered. "Everything is relative. You have to pick your path. To be honest with you, when I was working, 80% of the time I was really having a lot of fun and pleasant and exciting and thrilling. It was just 20% of the time that was very difficult and miserable and stressful. And, to me, that was the perfect ratio..."

# CHAPTER SIXTEEN

I was heading to my father's and planned to stop at a Japanese bakery called Ikeda's (where I'd discovered marionberry pies!) and asked if Sam knew of the bakery and if I could pick up something from him?

"Oh, yeah, we love marionberry," he responded, spiritedly. "Yes, we know and stop there often. We usually pick up a pie there…"

So, I purchased some items at Ikeda's and went to Sam's… And when Sam came to the door, I was taken aback by what I saw: Sam looked as though shrunken and significantly aged since the last time I'd seen him.

"I know it sounds dramatic, but it feels like this second bout of COVID-19 drained the life force right out of me," he said, breathless. "Just all of a sudden, you're lying there and it's hard to move up your arms, and breathing is really difficult."

But I didn't think he was being dramatic: It did look like the life force had been pulled out of him – everywhere!

"I don't know if a lot of it wasn't just the Covid accentuating the issues that I already had?" he continued. "Because when I'd start to exert myself, even before that second long Covid infection, I would feel that way, too. So, it wasn't entirely a new experience. It was just that that experience came on sooner. And the effects kept lingering, so that I didn't want to do anything.

"Before, it was my joints that were mainly messing up on me. My MCL. My torn hip. And I was recovering from that slowly, and building those muscles up stronger, using elastic bands and lifting weights and doing more range of motion exercises and stretching out. I was exercising before that. And I was getting there. Oh, Mike, I

**was doing so well! I was going, 'Oh, man, if I keep this up, I'm going to be better than I was when I was healthy.'**

**"And all of a sudden, when I got Covid, it just knocked me back so far, and I just couldn't do anything. I didn't want to do any of the exercises. Really, it was because I just couldn't. It was as if you had battery cells in every component of your body… In your arms and in your chest and in your hips and in your legs… And the batteries had all just run out of charge. They just ran out of charge everywhere.**

**"And I was thinking, 'OK, maybe I can't move my arm, but I should be able to move my leg.' But no, everything was just shutting down. It was like everything was drained..."**

## CHAPTER SEVENTEEN

Sam said his first bout of Covid had been difficult, but he had mostly recovered from that.

"I was doing really good," he said. "I was building up myself, and working on my muscles and my joints, and feeling really good, and coming back into strength, writing that bike, doing 1000 squats. And I thought, 'Oh, yeah, I'm going to be better and stronger than ever.' Then I got that Covid a second time, and it just wiped me out, and I've just been going downhill ever since."

He commented that his breathing difficulties actually began two or three years ago.

"I was taking that avalanche class," he said, "and I had to drop out of the final, because I just couldn't breathe up there when I was exerting myself, like skinning up the mountain. I barely made it up. And even a few years before that, I would just cramp up severely when I would go skiing. So, those were just initial signs that I was declining. But before the Covid, just doing average work or something, it was no problem. It was only when I would seriously exert myself. Then, I got this second Covid, and I just fell off the cliff..."

# CHAPTER EIGHTEEN

"In many ways, all the Covid did was accelerate my other issues," Sam contended. "But it was a major player in that. They say it affects your mitochondria. And it was systemic. It wasn't just my lungs. And I was having other issues, too. Psychological ones."

I asked why Sam hadn't told me before, especially given he knew I was having such good results in the Long COVID-Qi Gong study? He responded that it was because he'd been doing Qi Gong on his own since December.

"I do 20 minutes in the morning, and 20 minutes in the evening," he said. "And then I practice my tai chi forms when I can. And that's pretty much my exercise routine. Now that I'm not looking to do any running or skiing or riding my one wheel or electric unicycle or electric skateboard or roller skating.

"I was able to raise my minimal level of activity through proper breathing and things like that. But I wasn't actually reversing myself. All it was doing was improving a bad situation. It was sort of like, if you slept on your side, it would hurt and be uncomfortable. But if you move a slight bit, you would feel a little bit better. So, Tai Chi and Qi Gong exercises helps only in releasing the negative pressure slightly. It doesn't cure it. So, in a way it helps with the curing, but it's not the thing that cures it. It's sort of like the hospital has the vaccines or the antibiotics to help cure you, but the thing is, you've got to get to the hospital. Tai Chi and Qi Gong exercises get you closer to the hospital.

"So, the tai chi and the Qi Gong exercises were helping to position myself closer to get cured, but they don't cure you. They get you closer. So that you're like breathing better. It gives the opportunity for the immune system and your muscles to regenerate

**themselves properly. So, they're just fighting tiny battles, and some tactics are stalling and giving the opportunity to make things better..."**

# CHAPTER NINETEEN

Perhaps motivated by a desire to overcome my self-anger for missing or avoiding the clues that my friend was so ill (and I hadn't been helping him!), I pivoted to what Sam did best, and that was intellectually working through an issue, and I suggested we address the issue of his lack of energy by considering the question of long Covid as a mitochondrial illness as has been suggested?

What did that mean? I asked. Yes, mitochondria was essentially responsible for generating the key molecule for energy within cells (namely, ATP), but did that warrant calling long COVID a "mitochondrial disease"?

Sam agreed and considered the question.

"Is it the generating of ATP, or the recharging of the batteries, or both are damaged?" Sam conjectured. "You see, if you're battery can't accept anything, it doesn't matter about the ATP production. And if you're recharging is damaged, and your batteries are good, your batteries is not going to get charged. If both are damaged to certain degrees, they could have accumulative effect.

"So where are we? What do you try to fix? Are there ways to help boost the production of ATP? But if your battery is not able to accept it, it's like you're just running amuck with ATP.

"I would say in my situation, I don't think I'm making ATP. And if I have the capability of making ATP, the battery isn't charging.

"I don't even know if this analogy works for our systems. But that's the way our car works. Our car has a generator, and then it has a battery. And the battery activates the spark plugs. And an electric car works the same way, except that it has more batteries and more charging capacity. So, I imagine our bodies have a similar thing that reserve the ATP.

"Unless it's 'on-demand' ATP, so that whenever you need the ATP, the ATP is created by the mitochondria? But I would imagine there's a buffer system, which allows it to store it to keep things moving on an even keel. You don't want things to be spiking up, so that it's like, 'Yeah, I'm powerful, and now I'm weak. I'm powerful, I'm weak.' The body doesn't work with fluctuations very well. Drastic fluctuations; that is, 'Moments of inspiration, and moments of depression. Moments of inspiration, and moments of depression', 'I'm up, and I'm down. I'm down and I'm up'…"

Nevertheless, Sam thought it wasn't impossible that a virus could infect the mitochondria.

"The theory that every disease is related to an infection has not been disproven," he said. "But it hasn't been really proven, either. So that's just a nice academic paradox.

"But, in the long run, everything is in the web of life. Everything is related to one another in some form or fashion. To what degree and to when one is more relevant than the other, in certain illness states, who knows?

"Then, you have to ask, is it practical? Practical is to be able to say, 'Just give them this pill, and they'll be well.' Versus, 'Well, it's nice to know that about all of these things that can be underlying, but we don't know how to treat it.' Or, 'Well, we know how he died, but we couldn't save him.'

"And where does that come in with your practice of Qi Gong? Where are you on that spectrum? Are you really curing the person? Or were you just making them feel better, so that they can get an opportunity to cure themselves? And does it matter as long as the person in practical life becomes better? And all that is, is a probability game. Because if it just works for one or two people out of 100, is it worth the time to do that? Because you're wasting the time of 98 people to find the two people who it's going to help. Or does it help for 98 people out of 100, so that two people will be outliers? Because, then, it's very much worth it, because helping 98% of the time is phenomenal!"

It happened that in my Long COVID-Qi Gong study, the results were relatively 'phenomenal', and the 'outliers' were two participants who didn't perceive Qi, as those were the only two who didn't receive any benefit.

Meanwhile, I confided to Sam that when I shared the results of my Long COVID-Qi Gong study with the Chief of Medicine at the VA, he'd nonchalantly commented that he imagined that Qi Gong was a good and successful approach because long Covid represented a mitochondrial disease. In response, I thought, "How do you know that? How can you speak with so much certainty where that's concerned?

"Exactly," Sam commented. "I agree. It's a certainty until it's not. I mean, if it's the only thing you can grasp onto, then you grasp onto it. It's sort of like you're hanging off a cliff, and the only thing that you could hold onto is a piece of shrubbery. Do you hold onto it? Or not? And what's the chances of it de-rooting off the side of the cliff while you're holding onto it?"

He coughed heavily.

"In a situation like that, you can't see anything else," he continued. "There may be a really deep ingrained boulder that's barely sticking out that would be a great handhold and much more solid. But they don't see it. Because there's maybe dirt where it looks like there's no boulder there. But it's there - It's just not visible. So, you cling onto to your bush, which is actually de-rooting itself the longer you hold onto it.

"I know, because I've been there. And the problem is, something that you believe you're grasping on, like that bush and shrubbery, and then you put all of your hopes into it and all your weight into it, and then it just releases and you fall off the ledge.

"And it's psychological, too: When it comes to your Chief of Medicine and his sense of certainty and authority, it's because it's what he believes. Usually, people who say these things have an investment in it. Maybe it's what he's been preaching? Or feel that they have to go this route, where they don't get other people's approval?

"There's all kinds of stuff: If you dig down, you'll find out what the real reason is. And once you find out his real reason, then you have something to work with, and counter it.

"But, otherwise, you're just throwing things against the wall and hoping something sticks. You need to be more surgically precise, because it could be that what he's holding onto has a weak premise..."

# CHAPTER TWENTY

I thought about the spontaneous muscular releases that had been happening to me. For years, I'd wanted them to happen in my legs; but they'd concentrated in my torso, opening my chest to breath. Now, I wanted Sam to have the benefit of that.

I shared that this spontaneous muscular release process began happening after I started working with my father. That was back when I was doing the VA innovation accelerator project in 2022 and shared that video about Kino with my dad. My father asked if the kind of improvements that Kino was getting for his brain, might help with his brain, where he was having the difficulties of memory loss? I said I didn't know, but was willing to try. And the energetic experiences I had with my father I believe led to the imparting of these spontaneous muscular releases that have been the most important part of my personal healing ever since.

"That's really good that you felt that," Sam said of the spontaneous release experience.

Yes, I said, that certainly was a gift. A gift from my father - I suppose in exchange for the sacrifice in time and effort to see him every week.

I explained the way it happened: When I put myself in a supine, neutral position, the spontaneous muscular releases occur to mostly open up my chest.

"I think there's a lot to be said for being in a neutral position," he asserted. "Because then you're not putting tension and causing the body to skew. When the body does that, I think it can't feel things, because it's under tension somewhere. So, by un-tensioning everything, you have a better chance of realizing where there's a difficulty."

In this way I had my homework for the next days: Just as a drive to help Sam overcome his headaches five years ago had led to my being able to achieve Qi emission, I intended to apply that same drive to help Sam with this feeling of being drained.

In the meanwhile, performing external Qi Gong with Sam, I followed his energy outwards with my left hand, and it took me to my solar plexus - the energy center representing the seat of emotions.

This surprised me, because with all the discussion about 'drained batteries', if there were to be some chakra involvement, I was expecting a Dantian experience, because Traditional Chinese medicine holds that our energy reserve occurs there? But, no, for me it was the solar plexus. And maybe this made sense where Sam had previously told me he felt a lot of his issues were psychological?

"That's interesting that you were feeling it there," Sam commented. "I believe it's a good thing, because maybe you're getting closer to the root of it. I wish things were simple and straightforward, but I also feel that this type of thing requires maturity or evolution. Because in my situation, I'm feeling more and more weak. In my joints, I'm feeling the changes. I'm losing body mass."

"So, I'm changing, and therefore what you're feeling is a snapshot of my moment," he concluded. "And I'm changing all the time..."

# CHAPTER TWENTY-ONE

I called Sam from my father's and shared my stepmother's opinion that my father's dementia was a matter of 'God's design.' I, on the other hand, couldn't imagine God having any part of it. More, I remembered being a kid, and my father coming out of a restaurant and declaring it was full of "old people", and saying if he ever got that old, "to take me behind a barn and shoot me."

"Good thing you haven't found a barn," Sam inserted, humorously.

Then, during that visit, my stepmother nonchalantly called me over, saying my father was complaining about pain again, and asked me to help, because she was busy with some repairmen. I went walking over, thinking it was probably another cramp, like the hand cramp, then the leg cramp he'd had over the past days. But this time, it turned out the pain he was experiencing was in his chest!

Now, earlier that morning, he and I had been hard at work, shoveling snow off the driveway, so there was every reason in the world that he'd have pain from an intercostal or pectoralis muscle.

"Sure, he probably strained that muscle," Sam commented.

Yes, but I didn't want to take any chances and called an ambulance and had him taken to the hospital.

Still, there was the split second that the thought crossed my mind, "Maybe it wouldn't be the worst thing in the world if he was allowed to leave this earth with a heart attack and not continue to suffer all this frustration with his memory loss?"

"I understand what you're saying," Sam said. "And I think he probably has those thoughts, as well. Given I've been dealing with this thing [his health problems] for a long time, I've thought, 'What is a good way to die?' And then I realize that, for me, it's like going into a store where you can purchase a specific item or else you can buy the $25 'grab bag'.

With a $25 grab bag, there's usually more than $25 worth of merchandise when you've added it all up; but you don't know what's inside, so you don't know what you're getting: You might get something you like, so that you're pleasantly surprised and think, 'I would have never been able to get this at this price', or you might not.

"So, for me, when it comes to death, I think I went for the grab bag - I don't know how I'm going to die, but it's going to be more than what I paid for. And I don't know if I'm going to get 'quick and merciful' or 'slow and painful.' Instead, I got all these choices. With my luck, I'll get 'slow and painful.' I'll die in some foreign country jail - I'll be expedited over there, with my head shaved, and, for visual effects, tattoos put on me everywhere."

"You know, they could have done that to the Japanese," he added. "Rounded them all up and sent them to some country in South America. I mean, look, they were told: 'You're only allowed to take a suitcase with you, and you have three days to do it. And then we're gonna put you in some horse stables for temporary housing, and then we're gonna put you on a-train.' You know, you can compare it to the holocaust."

Yes, though, as my wife would say, here they weren't willing to go quite that far and "pull the trigger", as opposed to Nazi Germany, where they did.

"The point is, they didn't know what was at the end of their destination," he insisted. "It was like a simple version of the holocaust, in which you round up people and send them someplace.

"That's what they did today! They did that in this time! And they labeled them as 'gang members'. And maybe these people weren't the best of citizens, or average person who lives next-door to you, but they're human beings - Their people with lives. Who knows? They might have been your neighbor in 5 to 10 years. They might have been fantastic citizens. And yet they rounded these people up, with no due process!

"That's the thing – 'No due process.' They had no due process. In Germany, no due process. Now, in the United States.

"And they're doing it now. I don't understand how this can be? And then, to arrest a judge? A Judge? That's her courtroom. She should be able to do whatever she likes. She has that right. And it wasn't like she was deterring the ICE agents. She was essentially saying, 'If you want him, you'll have to do it outside of this court.' She was saying, 'You don't make an arrest in my courtroom.' I mean, it's a fine line, and a lot of people will say, 'Legally, she should not

**have done that.' But it's a fine line and couldn't you give the benefit of the doubt to the judge, who is in charge of that courtroom? The judge doesn't even do that to the accused. Because they're considered presumed innocent until proven guilty. They only do that when there's great concern that they need to be arrested, and I don't see the validation for a judge being treated that way. It was all just show. They could have just said, 'Judge, you know the law. you need to follow us, judge.' You give some decency to a public servant - the benefit of the doubt that way – to someone who's been divvying out the law for all of these years. Yet they give the president the leeway for criminal activity."**

**"So, we're talking about weird standards," he continued. "It's really tarnished our standing in the world.**

**"By the way, we're going to do to Greenland what Russia did to Crimea. And Canada is next. And then Mexico. Because we need a prison state. Will make Mexico into the prison state. Once we acquire Mexico, we'll send all of our 'bad hombres', as he would say, till we make Mexico into one big prison hell hole for the United States. Because, hell, we have so many criminals in the United States, and we only want certain kinds of criminals here - That we call 'Patriots.' We label these criminals, 'Patriots'..."**

# CHAPTER TWENTY-TWO

At the time, Pope Francis had just died, and the conclave was being assembled to elect a new Pope. Sam was saying that how Jesus would have lived and what he would have appreciated in a culture, rather than the ordinate lives of those leading the Catholic Church. I wondered that he would have appreciated the lives and spirituality of native peoples?

"Yes," he said, affected. "Yes. Actually, yes, in my opinion, he would have. And let's say Jesus wasn't born in Bethlehem, but instead he was born in New Mexico before it was part of the United States, and he introduced Christianity to the Native Americans. If that would have happened, the Catholic Church would look so much different."

Considering the thought of a Catholic Church with its origins in North America rather than Europe, I confided about how it was I heard stories about colonists, particularly colonist women, who, by choice, would leave the colonies to live among native peoples and how strange that struck me?

"Like, how could they have made such a choice?" I asked. "To live a life like that compared to what they had?"

"That's because you're brainwashed," Sam said, "to believe that they were savages. So, you were thinking, 'How could you choose to live like a savage? Why would you give up your wig and your fancy fluffy ruffled shirts, and not taking baths and putting on perfumes, for a life running around in a loin cloth, with sticks for weapons, and swimming in pools of water, and watching animals, and enjoying fresh air, instead of the sewers of London? Why would you give that up why? The stink of leather shops and leather manufacturing? Why

**would you give that up? Fucking-A? And all those hangings of people? Why would you give that up?'"**

**He hesitated.**

**"Yeah, I tell you, Michael, I think I would go for the Native American route. Walking the land and enjoying fresh air, eating fresh berries, having a nice barbecue. I tell you, Michael - Not a difficult choice..."**

# CHAPTER TWENTY-THREE

Sam posed questions about Energy Medicine and its practice.

"I was just wanting to understand your perspective and perception about people's ability when it comes to the energy to heal," he said. "Does it get stronger as they age? Or does it get weaker? Or do they need to practice it to maintain it? Is it a matter of, 'If you don't use it, you'll lose it'?

"Because what I want to know are questions like, Is it something that folks are born with? Does everybody have it? Does it come in different quantities? Does it come from the brain? They say your energy comes from your Dantian, which is around the belly button. So, where is your energy coming from? Or are you like a AAA battery, and you have this electrical charge throughout the whole thing? And if that's the case, if you lose a leg, are you less capable?..."

First, yes, I thought energy perception derived from the brain.

Second, yes, it was my understanding that Traditional Chinese Medicine teaches that the lower Dantian serves as an energy reserve to draw from in times of stress or trauma.

Third, regarding losing a body part, I wasn't sure what would happen to the overall energy of a person? Indeed, I wondered if it wouldn't actually enhance your energy perception ability because you had to rely more on your senses, and less on your physical being, not unlike what happened to me: I was struck by a car while riding my bike early in life; as a result, I couldn't do the physical things that I did before, and turned to more scholarly endeavors. I thought it would be the same with someone who, by some unfortunate circumstance, something happened so that they were less physically functional, and expected that they might become more energetically capable?

Sam asked if I'd seen Jasmine (my hairdresser, who I felt was an innate energy worker) and then pondered the question of why she could have been an energy worker?

"If these abilities to connect with the energetic circulation were stronger, why were they stronger in her than other people?" he asked. "Do hairdressers, in general, as an occupation draw certain people who have more ability that way? Because you never felt that type of experience with others, like in medical school. And here were with a group of people who want to be healers, and you were surrounded by them, and yet you didn't bump into any energy experiences with them that was significant enough to draw your attention. And here you are still with a group of healers - your current medical colleagues - and you don't seem to bump into a bubble of energy with them."

As for Jasmine, I just thought that she had some natural ability that came from her genetics and upbringing.

As for my medical colleagues, maybe it was because our western medical establishment is so violently opposed to energy medicine that people in the medical profession suppress any natural proclivity that way?

"So, there is a capability in people to lock it up?" he asked.

In general, yes, I thought that was the case, though there was Bill and Dr. K., who participated in the Qi Gong innovation accelerator project and performed Qi Gong so admirably and impressively.

And there was the time that a medical colleague (Dr. F.) who performed auricular acupuncture on me that triggered an energy experience, and I thought it was more than the needles that was involved.

"Could it be that people who perform eastern type of medicine practices have a better capability for connecting with the energy source?" he asked.

And connecting with other – Sure. Because, after all, eastern types of medical approaches, like acupuncture and other elements of traditional Chinese medicine were all about correcting the flow of Qi, so that it flowed in a more healthy manner, and, thereby, working at the individual physiology of the body, so to be more about facilitating the health of your individual patient.

"That gets back to my question of whether everybody has this ability to some extent?" he said. "But they either have to bring it out, or do they need to develop it? Or a combination of both? And do they have to use it, such that the more they use it, the stronger it gets?"

"That's what I'm hoping for you," he declared. "And that's why I think that whenever you get the opportunity, to use it. Because I imagine it's like most things, and you either use it or you lose it. And if you use it, you can grow it and nurture it more.

"And so, if that's the case, then a person in his or her first-year as a student, is going to become better at this as a second-year student, and then as a third-year student. Or in their fourth-year? You will see a growth, and you can plot it out, and maybe it reaches a saturation point? Or it will be exponential as it grows and continues to grow? You won't know until you are able to experiment with that."

"But then there's the question," he continued. "What would you use as an indicator for that? Is there one type of capabilities that would be an indicator for the rest of your Qi growth, so you use that as an indicator to show and plot out the Qi strength change?

"So much to think about. So much to learn and perform. But those are some of the things I think have to be performed.

"We know that it does something good. Your study has shown that. But they're still so little that we know about it and so much to do. It's like finding a little animal, and saying, 'I never knew that animal existed. But there it is. It's here.' But you don't know much about the animal: What will that animal look like a year from now? Or can I train it? Because, right now, everywhere it's unpredictable. Sometimes he's here, sometimes he's there. Sometimes it does remarkable things. Sometimes it just shits on you. It's just this little thing that you're chasing.

"But you know it's there. You say, 'It's there. I see it. It's on the ground. Sometimes when I corner it, I can work with it. And it provides me something. But what it's providing me and how it's providing it to me, I'm not sure? Can it provide me more?' Those are the things that I think about when I think about the things you're trying to do - I think it's like you're trying to chase this little guy..."

## CHAPTER TWENTY-FOUR

Thinking about Sam, I called April and shared about Sam's difficulties. In turn, she described her own struggles with long Covid.

"I had problems with long Covid for several years," she began, "and it was in the early days, and people didn't know so much about it, and I was just so fatigued.

"I was actually very diligent about reading all of the medical literature about long Covid, but I was keeping up with long Covid a lot, and I learned that, for some long Covid patients, the best thing was rest.

"And then that they discovered that there seems to be some damage to the mitochondria that's involved. So, when you say that Sam is very, very tired, I know that there's discussion about mitochondria damage and maybe he should look that up?

"Because when you had Covid, I tried to get permission from your doctor to give you time to rest. And then your doctor agreed with me and gave you a work excuse with a couple of weeks of total rest, and then six weeks of half days. And I think that made a difference for you…"

I called Sam and related April's comments. He mostly agreed.

"I felt my body needed rest," Sam responded. "And it's one of the most important aspects of getting better.

"And it wasn't like I had a choice, either: My body forced me to have rest, because I was just exhausted. It was like the worst case of malaise.

"But I think rest has to be supplemented with other things, and I haven't found what would help me accelerate beyond the rest? I know there's probably something out there, but I think it's also that I have a lot more complications with my health.

**"So, the Covid was kind of the last straw, and it just threw me off the cliff, so to speak. It's not just my long Covid, but also my other issues, and what's gonna help me with all of them? And which one is more dominating? Or which one is causing more synergistic effects?**

**"So, it's like kind of like trying to fight a battle or a war, with many fronts… You're being attacked at all sides, and it's kind of hard to put your emphasis on how to get better, because you're being distracted in all areas."**

**"So, in my case, I'm different," he declared, "and it would be nice if long Covid was the only thing I had to deal with."**

**"Anyways, I just have to figure out ways to improve my situation," he concluded. "So, I'm experimenting with all kinds of stuff - Supplements and exercise and activities…"**

## CHAPTER TWENTY-FIVE

Calling Sam again, he described problems with his throat.

"Some people call it a tickle in your throat," he began. "I call it a splinter in my throat. That's what it feels like. It's like as if I had a sliver there. Or a splinter in my throat. And I'm trying to cough it up. It's like you ate some cactus, and the needles are stuck in your throat. And there's no coughing them out.

"And I feel all wound up, because I'm trying to hold back my coughing, and you know how it is to hold back a sneeze?... Well, that's how it feels - In my whole body. My head, shoulders, chest. Especially my chest. I'm holding it back because I don't want to cough. Just trying to stop multiple things at one time…"

Hearing this, I lost it and couldn't bear my friend suffering this way, and told my father and stepmother that I was heading back early to try to help my friend...

## CHAPTER TWENTY-SIX

Arriving at Sam's, I told him that I wanted to take him through an experiment. First, I stated the hypothesis: I had told him that my internal Qi Gong practice had moved to spontaneous muscular releases, usually occurring throughout my torso, so that it was bang, bang, bang, bang, bang when it came to these muscular releases, opening me up at my shoulders, ribcage, back, and even solar plexus. What's involved in that? I think it's some kind of unhinging of the actin and myosin fibers that were holding the muscles in a state of permanent contraction and spasm.

"You release the ratchet," Sam offered, insightfully. "Because it's ratcheting… Click, click, click, click… and contracting till you release it."

Right, I said. That's exactly what's occurring. But it seems to me that at the initiation of that release mechanism required some source of charge, and I held that was some quality of Qi that my father had imparted to me, so to reactivate my self-repair mechanisms for that; and now I was going to try to impart something akin to that to Sam, so as to attempt to reactivate his energy producing mechanisms.

We had Sam lay on the floor (in the way that I did when I underwent the muscular releases), and from there, I'd attempt Qi Gong on him.

As I connect with him energetically, Sam described experiencing bubbles, popping gently in his muscles, and allowing them to elongate.

"I feel this pop, and then I feel relaxed," he said. "Like there's this air bubble there, and it goes pop, pop, like I'm pressing on a bubble pack. And it's very distinct. I can feel it in the lower calf area and ankle above the Achilles tendon, and then all along both arms.

**"I didn't feel that in my chest, but I felt relaxed. Like I felt normal - With no issues - And I'm not feeling anything in my throat, either."**

**"I tell you, Mike," he concluded, "I think it was a good thing for me to have you do that..."**

# CHAPTER TWENTY-SEVEN

As Sam didn't have the same experience that I did, I decided to attempt to show him the spontaneous muscular releases that happen with me when I perform my Qi Gong self-practice.

Laying on the floor, I put myself in a Qi Gong state and immediately experienced a muscular release that lifted me off the carpet.

"It looked like it came from your spine area," Sam commented.

Yes, I agreed. It felt like that release had come from my mid to lower back.

"So, it's just relaxing muscles that just seem to be a little tight?" he deduced.

He said he'd had similar experiences.

"There are times that I'll feel my arm just jerk," he said. "It will typically surprise me, and I'll go, 'Whoa, what was that?'"

Yes, it sounded like essentially the same kind of process that I was experiencing, except his system was doing it automatically, without his having to put himself in a Qi Gong state; and, for whatever reason, working with my father had facilitated this self-repair system that others (like him) took for granted; and now I was perhaps catching up with everybody else, and that's why I was having muscular releases that lifted me from the floor, whereas his amounted to the popping of air bubbles?

"You're making up for lost time," he commented...

## CHAPTER TWENTY-EIGHT

Departing, Sam escorted me to my car.

"I'm going to tell you, I think my lung thing is more than just Covid," he said, "because I was getting more short of breath before Covid. It's just that Covid just threw me off the cliff. Before, I was just getting close to the cliff, and all of a sudden, Covid just threw me off."

We would throw him back on, I thought. We'd recharge his system and perhaps that would be the catalyst to help him with his shortness of breath all by itself?

But then the bottom seemed to fall out the next day: As April and I were walking in the orchards of Village Homes, admiring the apricot and cherry trees in full bloom and near ready for foraging, Sam called.

"Mike, I thought I should inform you that I just got out of an appointment with my Pulmonologist," he said. "She said that my interstitial lung disease has advanced, so that I probably don't have long to live. She says I qualify to be a lung transplant candidate, but first I have to get a lung biopsy."

I stood stunned. Here we were making headway and a possible breakthrough where figuring out how Qi Gong might get Sam past the problems of long Covid and massive fatigue and lack of energy and potentially recharging his mitochondria, and now he was being told that he had an irreversible, untreatable lung condition that was going to kill him!

"It's most likely that I'll pass away in my sleep," he continued. "I think that's what it will probably come down to. I'll fall asleep and it will end.

**"It's like the frog in the beaker, and all of the sudden, it's reached that point, and then it's not able to wake up.**

**"I think it's a long way off yet. But I feel so tired, and I just want to sit down - lay down - and rest.**

**"And I know that that's a prelude that it will just progress really bad, until there's not much we can do.**

**"I just hope I get a lot of things done before that. So, I'm working on my income tax now. So, my accountant will be happy..."**

# CHAPTER TWENTY-NINE

Returning to Sam's, we talked about his condition. As air hunger was my worst fear in life, I couldn't imagine anyone not being overcome with dread and anxiety over the prospect of it?

"You get used to it," Sam asserted. "I'm getting used to it. The first time, it's always fearful. You think, 'What's happening?' And it feels painful, too - because it's a new sensation. But, then, afterwards, like everything else, you get kind of used to it. And all the sudden you go, 'Yeah, I'll get out of this. I can hold on.' Or, 'It's not as frightening', and it becomes a familiar situation."

"It's interesting," he added, philosophically. "Everyone is going to go through what I'm going through now. Unless someone comes up to you and shoots you in the head, it's going to happen. It's like a dream, and you start to wake up, and it's like no time went by. It's just like everything unfolds.

"I always wondered when a little baby is born and it passes away in five minutes or whatever, I keep thinking, 'Within that five minutes – That was a lifetime for that child. What is actually going on? What is a life for them? What is a five-minute life for a child who is born and then passes away? What is that lifetime like? Is it much different for someone living for close to 100 years old?' Because, in the end, I don't see that person really thinking like we're thinking right now.

"The people who passed away when I was right there… Well, their thoughts and conversations were nothing even close to the way that we're talking about it now. It's if they were just born and passed away within minutes of their birth. The person who is passing away in the bed… Well, some people think that they whisper things, like their loved ones' names and things like that. And they may do that. But what's actually going through the minds of those people?

"Just like we say about God… What do we really know of God? At the end, when we're about to report to God, they say that every person turns religious when they're dying. But just because they say God's name at the end, what does that really mean? Are they just grasping onto the last lifeline? Was it really a grasp? Or was it just them fading away and the only thing that they could think of and their last neural activity was something to do with death, and God is there, especially when it comes to an afterlife."

"I just want to focus on the good things," Sam concluded. "That's why I got the sewer fixed. That way, I don't have to be bothered about the sewage coming back up, and that I've made it comfortable for May in the house. It's costing us a lot of money to get rid of the asbestos in the house; the thing is, though, Mike, I just want to live a comfortable life. That's why we did this landscaping - So, I can sit here and talk with people I care about, and we can have nice little conversations and enjoy.

"I'm just wondering about how debilitated I'm becoming? Because this Saturday we're going to go on a hike at Putah Creek. Really, it's not a hike; it's kind of a nature walk. There's gonna be a lot of stopping, so I should be able to handle it. And I've got to do some exercise. And that's why it was nice that we walked in the park the other day, from bench to bench."

As Putah Creek was near Davis, I asked if I could come and support him?…

# CHAPTER THIRTY

Arriving home, April commented that she thought Sam would be regarded as a "found family brother" by the Lakota.

"I was thinking about [Prof.] Albert White Hat's book, Zuya, where he talks about, in the Lakota tradition, there is 'found family' - the brothers who you choose. And I was thinking that Sam was a brother you chose. And that Lakota Brothers were just as important as the family that you're born into... He is your Lakota brother..."

Calling Sam, he talked about the instruction he'd received in Tai Chi and Qi Gong over the past year.

"One good thing about this situation and my condition is that it has made me really sensitive to proper form in my biomechanics and my breathing and my whole body working properly," he said. "So, it's really interesting that I'm finding that my condition helps me get better [at Tai Chi and Qi Gong], because it indicates when I'm doing things wrong."

He coughed terribly.

"Anyway, that's one thing I've discovered," he continued, "and I've never felt this level of fine tuning of my movements."

I commented that when everything flows, it's referred to as being in a Qi Gong state.

"Oh, yeah, I truly believe that," he responded. "I think that's where Qi Gong wants you to be. It's about letting go.

"There are people who say, 'Oh, I do Qi Gong. I do Tai Chi.' But they're making the movements, but do they really feel it? I mean, they feel something. When I first started, I could feel this tingling, and I thought, 'Oh, I must be doing it right.' And then, as I did more and more of it, I got more of that tingling, and I realized that that tingling is moving towards it [Qi Gong state], but it's only being halfway or a quarter of the way there.

"And I think that's the thing that I see in the videos when people do this. They profess in the videos that they're doing Qi Gong and Tai Chi and all this, but I keep thinking, 'I think you guys are making your video premature.' But then, I find other people, and I think, 'Oh I think they're doing it so good.'

"So, for me, I'm always my best subject. It's like my ski deck: The more I practice on it, the better I feel and the more it becomes effortless and just seems like, 'God, everything just works.'

Yes, that was always what I saw when I watched him ski – A ski sensei - effortlessly, magically, gliding and flying through the snow…

I commented that the goal of Qi Gong was to bring it so much into your life that at every moment you were in that Qi Gong state.

"Yes, I'm not there yet," he responded, breathless. "But I'm working towards it.

"But I can tell you this… My stress on my chest and throat and my circulation and getting lightheaded and all that is starting to become more prominent. And the thing is, when I'm doing Qi Gong and feeling like I'm doing it pretty properly, it just flows.

"And it's amazing. I always say, at the beginning of this form is like slowly riding a bike uphill. I have to work at it. But once I get to a certain point, every form after that seems like they're connected, and I'm riding downhill.

"And also I notice my movements speed up. Like it's slow at the beginning, and then once I get to a certain point it feels effortless."

He went through the names of the different Tai Chi movements.

"And all that seems to move very smoothly, like I'm riding downhill, and linking each one, so it seems like one leads right into the next one, so it feels so effortless.

"And my breathing isn't hard, so it feels really good. In fact, my breathing is more in sync and it feels so comfortable.

"Oh, Mike, I feel like a little kid, riding down a mountain road, going downhill, with my mouth open, and feeling the rush of air, and my hair flowing back, and my legs are just effortlessly peddling the bike. And it's a really neat feeling..."

# CHAPTER THIRTY-ONE

Sam's description of feeling like a kid peddling on a bike while doing Tai Chi and Qi Gong reminded me of the way he always was on the slopes – Smiling and laughing, as he carried his skis around, slung over his shoulder, talking with people, and having a great time...

Sam went on about working with Tai Chi instructors with 40 years-experience.

"I'm only three months into it, but what my goal is, Mike, is to work 30 years, from now until I pass away, which can be a very few months, or it could be a couple of years or whatever, who knows? I'm trying to cram into a few months, several decades of tai chi practice.

"Because I did the same thing with skiing. A lot of people said I couldn't do that, but, of course, I had the ski deck, and that accelerated my skill development tremendously. And so, it's one of those things that I kind of say, 'What's my ski deck for Tai Chi? How do I do that?' And I developed a program for myself to try to do that in my stricken situation.

"Because I can't be just practicing Tai Chi. I can only do this form two or three times at the longest, because I just can't last. And sometimes I could only do it one time for the whole day.

"And yet I have developed one-third of a 30-year practice crammed in this timeframe. I kind of figured out how to do it, but it's just a little bit complicated to explain. But it seems to be working, even when I can't do much of it during the day.

"And I think this is the way that a lot of masters of Qi Gong did this, because I think when they learned the basic forms, they were able to adapt.

"It's sort of like a musician: Once they learn how to play a few songs, but do it really, really well, like Beethoven's Sonata, and that's all they practice… Well, then, all of a sudden, they're able to pick up any music sheet and play it really well right away."

"It's like trying to develop the secret of life, so to speak," he concluded, "and I'd like to accomplish that for mind body things."

As he spoke, I thought about my book writing: My first book, I made over a thousand modifications before I was ready to let it go to publication; now, I was putting out books much faster, and, to my surprise, even my author friends indicate they're happy with the quality of the writing.

"Yes, exactly," Sam said. "It's similar. The person who knows how to do that really well is the person who studies: 'What were the steps that made me get so good eventually on my first book?' And then try to adopt those things into their second book. And then learn more things that help and do it on their third book. And it's those people, who do those things, who become true masters and have developed it.

"And it really takes a lot of thought. Maybe for some people, it's easier, but I had to make a lot of mistakes to continue to develop.

"In a way, I feel very, very grateful for the condition I'm in. Because if I was really healthy, there wouldn't have been any motivation to do any of this. In fact, if I was really healthy, I wouldn't have done Tai Chi at all. As I was growing up, I always felt Tai Chi was kind of a silly thing to do. And Qi Gong was silly. I felt like, 'I don't want to do Tai Chi. I don't want to do Qi Gong. I don't have the time. I have no need for it. I'm healthy. I can do things. There wasn't any need for that.' It's only when I get this illness that that changed."

"That's why I always say, the bad things – the worst things – that have happened in my life have been my greatest teachers…"

# CHAPTER THIRTY-TWO

Sam continued, describing his previous disregard for Tai Chi and Qi Gong.

"In fact, when I was younger, in my mind, I used to tease [those performing Tai Chi and Qi Gong]. I never said it out loud, but I used to think, 'Damn, that's such silly movements. I wouldn't be caught dead trying to do those things.' when I was young and healthy and strong and felt like I knew what the world was all about. So, it's really such a complete turnaround for me.

"And that's the way a lot of Trump people are: They feel strong and healthy, and they don't want to listen to a lot of other people with problems, because they don't feel like they have the problems. And so why should they be concerned?..."

I asked Sam about how it was that his previous illness (with the hypopituitary and hypothalamic condition) didn't urge on all of these same things, as compared to what he was going through now? Why would that not have promoted the same "sensitivity" as an illness?

"That was a different type of sensitivity," he asserted. "You know, the body is very complex in my opinion. And my mind is also very limited, too – Narrowminded, with blinders on. It gave me some, but it left out many others.

"I'm going to tell you: One thing doesn't solve everything else. It's like these people who are experts at one thing, and then they go into politics, and they think they're experts on everything – like it's the same thing. When, no, it's like, 'You're really, really good at this focus area, but you're not good in other areas. Until you put the time in, and effort, and have the passion for it.'

"So, for me, there is a relationship [to his hypothalamic illness], but it's not a very strong one."

"It did give me weakness," he explained. "I'm going to tell you, that felt more like Covid - The weakness I felt. Because without that testosterone, I felt really weak.

"But, as you know, the cause of it is totally different than long Covid. It's not the same. One is testosterone hormone levels. The other one is ATP levels. That's probably very crude and there's more involved than that, but the basics are different in my opinion. And so, I had to deal differently with that, then I am with this."

He described what it was like to have to receive testosterone replacement therapy.

"When I took too much testosterone, I was aggressive, nervous, my temper was short, and I wouldn't dwell on the issue that I was facing," he said. "And I've always been someone who is calm, cool and collected.

"So, I really wound up understanding women and how their menstrual cycles affect them. I was really sympathetic to women and their mood swings after my testosterone thing…"

After a fit of coughing fit, Sam elaborated about his deteriorating health.

"My knees and my hip," he said. "I'm a total mess. But I'm livable with myself. It's been like this for many, many years now. But now things have gone worse because of the lungs.

"Everything is getting a little bit worse. It's sort of like I'm watching myself and then imagining myself just falling apart."

He talked about his worsening skin condition.

"I've got scars everywhere on my body," he began. "I can't even be taking off my shirt because I'm looking like a leper from a leper colony.

"So, there's a lot of things I'm facing all at one time. I'd never wish anybody to be like me. But I'm just making deal with what I have and what I can do. And I'm still going to make a full life while I can live.

"When it gets to a point that I'm bedridden or I lose my ability to think, or if I get stuck in a wheelchair, then things get pretty serious. Because I'm really limited then.

"Even my taste I sort of lost with Covid. It's only been a month or so that I've regained my taste and been able to eat more. So, I'm starting to eat now more and enjoy flavor. That's why I sort of just go out and buy what I want."

"I'm just letting you a little bit into my life," he concluded. "I tell

**people, 'Don't worry about me, because I'll make do and I'll still enjoy, until I can't.' I'll do everything until I can't…"**

# CHAPTER THIRTY-THREE

Sam called the following day, saying that he was "going downhill fast."

"It's so difficult to get up and to breathe," he began, "and I'm getting signs with my left arm, falling asleep a lot, and recovery is really hard. And then this morning, I kind of soiled myself a little bit. So now I'm losing bladder control. And that's the first time that's something like that happened. And I just thought, 'This isn't good.'

"I'm losing muscle. And also, I try to do tai chi yesterday, and I just kind of lost my balance and wasn't able to get it as smoothly as I had before, and I can tell that even with Tai Chi, which isn't very strenuous, it's hard for me to move my body parts. And it's amazing how this is all happened over a short amount of time?"

He indicated it was only a few months ago that he'd passed his breathing tests, and last week, he didn't.

"So, I'm feeling like it's just a matter of a short amount of time before my lungs are not going to be able to function at all," he said. "So that I think the lung transplant is all I have.

"But the main reason why I called was, while I was still lucid, I was wondering if you would help guide May through my last days?" he asked. "Helping to explain things to her - definitely from the medical side.

"Because May will be wondering, too, if she could have done something that would have prevented this. She's always insisted I take aloe vera and thought of these little things. I haven't complied with a lot of them, but I thought it was nice, and I thought it might have helped a little bit, but not in the long run.

"So, things like that. And her guilt - It will be important to give her a view from a medical standpoint about my situation. And then I might need you to look at my medical records and see what I might have done differently. That would be helpful for someone else."

"Just a little bit," he continued. "Because there's no one who knows me more and my conditions than you."

He hesitated.

"I was always hoping that my lungs would heal a little bit," he continued. "But I doubt it now..."

## CHAPTER THIRTY-FOUR

"Yesterday was the toughest day I ever had," Sam continued. "And that was because I had four visitors. And it taxed me, because I was trying to be as strong as I could: I taught a lesson and that was really, really wonderful; and then, two former students came, and I gave them some equipment that they wanted, like some waxing stuff, and talking with them and trying to find that equipment was really taxing; and then, the fourth person was a friend for whom it's been something of a mixed bag… Really good guy, but he asked for some stuff, and it took so much out of me. Afterwards, I was just sitting there trying to recover, and my recovery time is getting really, really long, versus before when all I had to do was sit down for a while.

"I need to figure out how I can get you access to my medical records. I don't want to burden you, but it might be that I'll hallucinate something, because now everything that doctors tell me go into one ear and out the other; because my filtering system is getting fogged up; so I can't make quick decisions, and correct decisions.

"I think May is understanding my situation quite a bit, but I just feel like I needed to let you know where I was at.

"Anyway, today I'm going to try to be as normal as possible and try to catch up with financial records and clean up and clear up as much as I can. But I think it's just a good relief to tell somebody."

I asked if I could help?

"No, I think it's good for me," he responded. "I think if I don't do something, I feel like I'll be a burden to others, and that adds to my stress levels, though sometimes I wish I had an extra pair of hands that would help me.

"I just want to get some things cleared up. Definitely, there are some big things on my mind, like the sewer line getting filled in properly. I know I'm talking little stuff here, and I'm not trying to avoid my big issue, but this all has an effect on my mind. Like, for instance, putting back the dirt. It's not all going to be able to be put back in, and I don't know what to do with the rest of the dirt? The people from the city dumped gravel so that the lines wouldn't be exposed, but it filled half of the hole, so now there's all this extra dirt. And if we scatter it through the yard, it just messes up the yard.

"So, maybe there's someone who will pick up the excess dirt and haul it away somewhere? I don't know. But things like that bother me and create a burden on my mind, because that just leaves something that my family has to deal with.

"I know I shouldn't be worried about that, but sometimes the pressure of the mind is so much greater than the physical pressures. So, it's something that's distracting me that shouldn't be, but yet it burdens me. So, it's little things like that that I have to take care of, so they won't be burdening my mind."

I asked if I could load the dirt in my truck and haul it away for him?

"That's a very good idea," he said. "We just need to find a place to unload it. Let's see how much dirt is remaining after we backfill it. I don't want to keep impinging on you, because you've done so much for me. Let's take it one step at a time. But that is something that's bothering me. And now that we've talked it through, I don't feel so bad, because there's an outlet for it and things can get done."

I raised the issue that I didn't understand why his doctor was only talking about lung transplant, and not raising other treatments with medications like antibiotics and corticosteroids, inhalers and immunosuppressants? It just seemed like there were a lot of other treatments to be considered? And here he was yet to have a biopsy, so it didn't seem his diagnosis was nailed down?

"I don't know," he replied, wearily. "It could be that it's my fault and a lot of this stuff suddenly happened, too. I think she did say something about treating me with corticosteroids, but thought that a biopsy would be important to perform first."

I'd previously given him some papers about his condition and asked if we shouldn't go over them today?

"Yeah, that would be good," he said. "It would be nice to know. And I didn't to read it, because I haven't had a chance to catch my breath, so to speak..."

# CHAPTER THIRTY-FIVE

"I wanted to show you my Tai Chi form," Sam continued, "but I tried to do it for May last night, and it was kind of wobbly, and I was going, 'My God?! A few hours before that, I felt really solid, and, all of a sudden, I lost it.' Now, is that the immune process? Or is my body just giving out? I don't know."

I asked if he thought it could be due to his lungs and oxygen levels?

"Oh, yes," he said. "I think that is probably it. I think I can't maintain my oxygen saturation in my condition. I think my whole body is competing for that little amount of oxygen that's there. That's why I cramp up easily. And my muscles feel kind of weird now. Because when I use them, it uses up that oxygen, and it taxes all my other systems.

"At rest, I'm at 95%, but once I start moving around, I imagine it drops. Well, it did - It dropped during the six-minute [breathing] test."

I suggested that we go to Stanford and get him a second opinion from the lung experts there?

"Sam, the way things are going, I think either you're going to wind up in a local hospital and just take whatever they can give you," I said, "or else you can get in my car and I'll drive you to the ER at Stanford, where they probably have some of the best lung experts in the world.

"It's not quite there I don't think," he asserted. "But soon. Definitely. I'm going to drop off here.

"What happens is, I work a little bit here, and then I rest and try to recover. And if I pace myself, I can last for a long time.

**"But then we could talk about all that if you are going to make it out here."**

**I told him that I was getting on the road now.**

**"Mike, take your time," he said. "Don't worry. I've got to try to get my morning going and eat breakfast and all that. Take your time..."**

## CHAPTER THIRTY-SIX

As I went to the car, April voiced her support for my assisting Sam, saying she was living vicariously through my doing all the things for Sam that she wished she had done for her friend, Robert.

"It's such an honor that he's letting you in to this moment," she said.

Sadly, after I arrived at Sam's, he said didn't have a lot of time, because he had to get to a family gathering.

"My aunt is coming," he said, "and that's going to be very important, so I'm going to try to build up my energy..."

He wanted to show me a Qi Gong video made by Qi Gong master he'd been learning from over the past six months.

"It's a 20-minute video," Sam said. "I want to do it every day. I began doing it because I thought, 'There's got to be something to it, or else why would Dr. Mike dedicate so much of his time to it?'"

"You helped me grow in it," he added. "So, I thank you very much..."

After watching the video and before he left for the family gathering, I insisted we talked about Stanford. I told him that my experiences with Stanford had been exceedingly good. For example, when my father was diagnosed with a Schwannoma of the brain, his Carson City specialist recommended immediately gamma-knife surgery; but I convinced my father to get a second opinion at Stanford first, and when we went there, the Stanford specialist calmly laid out the options for my father, saying that most people with his condition don't experience significant growth of the tumor, and it can be safely watched with serial MRIs every six months, so that most likely he was not going to require surgery, which can only be performed once via gamma knife, and then, if it has to be done again, will involve extensive neurosurgery; and with that expert advice, my father avoided an unnecessary procedure.

I continued that, in Sacramento, Sam had been dealing with a Pulmonology group with doctors coming and going, telling him different things, and now he sees this new Pulmonologist for the first time, and she's telling him that he needs an open lung biopsy and lung transplant on the first visit. To me, it sounded just like my father's experience in Carson City, with the specialist there telling him he needed to go under the gamma-knife, and the folks at Stanford rightly telling him he didn't; and maybe we'd have some luck and find the same at Stanford for him.

Sam raised the issue of that going to Stanford meant a two-hour car ride. I responded by telling him about my experience during my residency in Los Angeles. When I worked between LA County General Hospital and Martin Luther King Hospital, I expected I see the same kind of pathology between the two hospitals, because both were serving essentially the same population.

But I was wrong - Because the people in Compton and Watts might not have had a lot of wealth, but they could usually beg, borrow or steal $30, and that was enough for a taxi ride to LA County; and there was a general recognition within the Southcentral LA population that if you had a serious medical condition that required a bit more diagnosing than you could get at MLK, then you paid the extra $30 and got yourself to LA County.

"They called it '$30 sick'," I said, "and it seemed to me that you've reached that threshold, and it's time to put in the extra time and money to go to Stanford, and I'll personally take you."

"I hadn't thought about it in those terms," Sam responded. "But I certainly will and get back to you..."

## CHAPTER THIRTY-SEVEN

During the night, Sam reached out to me, saying that he was feeling worse, and when he shared my idea of taking him to the Stanford ER with a cousin who was a doctor, his cousin agreed and that really tipped the scale.

"That surprised me," he said, "because my cousin doesn't usually agree with me about a lot of things, especially medical ones."

"The one piece of advice he gave me," he added, "was to get there early…"

We left for the Stanford ER at about six in the morning. As we drove, we talked about Yale, and I relayed a conversation that I'd had with April about where I do and don't thrive.

*"You don't thrive under harsh treatment and conditions," April had said. "You thrive when people are warm to you and encouraging. And you need a person that you can be complaining, and they'll value you enough to deal with it. Because you need to complain, or else I think you get triggered, and then you trigger others."*

And at Yale, there was a pretty tough lady (Dr. Patrika) who had been selected to serve as my mentor, and I was afraid she was going to be harsh.

"Dr. Patrika might not be warm and supportive and enthusiastic," Sam responded, "but maybe this represents an opportunity for you to realize that these people do exist in the world, and you getting to do work that you have a passion for might get you through this kind of difficulty, so that you can learn and figure out how to work with folks like this?

"You say, 'I have a passion that gave me the motivation to figure out and say, "OK, I'm being beaten, but I have to figure out an out here, and all of the sudden I'll come up with it. And it's only because I have a passion for it, and I love it, and I've studied it in and out. And I don't have all the answers, but I know what makes me happy. And I got people who are up against me. But I always find a way to overcome them. Because I realize that they have weaknesses".'

"And maybe you'll find that they just had the wrong idea about you. And they don't know you. They just think they know you - They've already pictured who you are. They've already developed a strategy for you. Because they show it so clearly. They think that you're incompetent and unable to do it yourself. And they said right out loud to you by thinking bad about you. So, they think that you can't do those things.

"It's like, when you're dealing with a child, you make presumptions about what this child is and what their capabilities are. And so, you start emphasizing things. And the child gets really frustrated. He thinks, 'I know how to do this. And you're just over killing me. You're making things worse. And if you just left me alone, I would figure it out and do it.'

"And so, to me, they're treating you like a child. And you know what? They probably have a habit of that. Because, guess what? They've been dealing with young graduates, who think they know how to do things and they don't.

"You, on the other hand, have gone through this. Look at all your credentials - They're ignoring them. In fact, they're probably saying this: 'Why is this doctor leaving his practice? Maybe he's not that good? And that's why he wants to do this?' They're characterizing you.

"So, I think you need to look at it where they're coming from, and maybe then you can see why their behavior towards you is the way it is. I think you have enough confidence now to know that you're going to make it work.

"They're expecting you to fail. But yet they're taking a chance on you, saying, 'Well, maybe there is something to it? To his approach?' And that's why they're being so strict on you, and treating you like a child.

"And you have the chance to succeed. Just think, if you can overcome this and these people, you can overcome the world.

"So, I think this is an opportunity. And the only way you're going to see this as an opportunity is when you have it behind you. And the only way you're going to have it behind you if you go to walk into the fray..."

"Anyway, Mike," Sam continued, "if they thought that you were totally worthless, they would not even have had you come on board. Someone is fighting for you."

Yeah, I said. Ellen.

"And I think you should show her that her judgment is a really good judgment that you will come through for her and your success will come through like an overspray."

He hesitated.

"I don't know, Mike," he concluded. "It's hard. You could try to go the cautious route, but the cautious route will cause you to miss an opportunity. Again, it all falls on your decision…"

# CHAPTER THIRTY-EIGHT

I confided that among my apprehensions was what if the patients at Yale were different than those in California, and the hardy New Englanders there weren't interested in Qi Gong or able to perceive it at all? After all, I was entering a totally different culture that I really didn't know anything about it. I had never worked in New Haven. What if they looked at what I was doing like it was voodoo?

"But don't you think that the people in your [UC Davis] study might have had thoughts like that, too?" Sam asked.

Yes. Indeed, none of the folks in the study had any experience with Qi Gong, and from the first group until the last, they described disheartening experiences, in which people in their lives questioned their sanity for participating in the study.

"Right," Sam said. "I would think that these people in Connecticut might be a little bit more stubborn. But just like you won them over here in California, I think and I hope that that will be the least of your worries. And if you find that you really focus on doing the best you can, and not worrying about their opinions, then you'll come up with the same results. Or very similar."

Yes, based on past experience, probably the most significant thing I had to be afraid of was my self-sabotaging the study.

"Yeah, I tell you, there's a lot of pressure on you," Sam responded, compassionately. "Let the cards show what they show. There's nothing that you can do. Even the negative results will teach you something. You'll be able to say, 'Oh, I see what I did.' And the only way that you can do it and not feel intimidated is by not being discouraged by negative results.

"I was watching a documentary in which successful people… Well, even they went through a time that things did not work out. And they were trying to problem solve, and asking, 'What did I do wrong?' And that's what makes it exciting. It's the overcoming of a weakness or failure."

We passed the wooded Stanford powwow grounds along a beautiful meadow lined with eucalyptus trees. I thought about the many years that I served native peoples as an Indian Health Service physician on Indian Reservations of the Northern Plains. The native healers and Medicine Men there had intuited my abilities and appreciation for "energy healing" and appreciated that I'd been initiated in Qi Gong and quickly introduced me to their ceremonies and shared their ways. Where there was once a hint of a suspicion that I might have come to "convert" the people there, that was quickly perished, as it was obvious that I was the one who was "converted." There ways had become my ways, and I could do nothing but bow to their superior spirituality and still long for the feeling of peace I found on the Reservations.

"But, Mike, you can't be a one hit wonder," Sam declared. "The only way you can keep from doing that is by pursuing it. And you can do it.

"So, what's the worst-case scenario? You go to Yale and it totally flops. And you realize that the successes that you had in the past were flukes. This is the worst scenario. The worst of the worst. Then you would say, 'You know what? I learned that it doesn't work. So, I'm now going to focus my life on what does work, instead of continuing to pursue something that doesn't.' OK? That's the very, very worst. But you would have proved it to yourself that it doesn't work.

"Now, I don't think that's going to happen. You are going to find something that's positive. And the positive could be small, it could be medium, or it could be large. And if you position it properly, it could be very large.

"I think going to Yale, you're going to be able to define the power of this. You might find things that are frustrating to you, but I think you're gonna come out of it with something wonderful."

"You've shown it works," he concluded. "So, you just need to define that. I think it all just comes back to my original thought that you should be damn proud."

At that moment, we arrived at the Stanford Emergency Department...

# CHAPTER THIRTY-NINE

Perhaps because it was Mother's Day, the waiting room for the Emergency Department was mostly empty. After checking in at the front desk, a nurse set about taking Sam's vital signs. Despite being mostly business-like, she did take the time to inquire about the meaning of Sam's surname.

"It means, 'Forest Island'," Sam responded, kindly.

The nurse nodded her, nonchalantly. Then, she noted the results of Sam's oxygen saturation and straightened.

"Are you very short of breath?" she asked.

Indeed, even as we'd parked the car, Sam had indicated that he was surprised at how short of breath he felt.

After a short conversation between the nurse and the front staff, Sam was taken back into the main part of the Emergency Room, with plans to admit him to the hospital…

As we waited and different Emergency Department staff came in and out, Sam talked about the Qi Gong master in the video.

"Did you notice how he talked?" he asked. "About the energy flowing through your spine? He adds these things with the movements, so you can relate with the feeling. And I guess what I'm saying is that you do the same thing. And they're feeling it. That's the only reason why these people would remember it. They say, 'Yeah, I hear it, I feel it.' Just like the way a good Qi Gong master works with Qi. That's why I think Nolan is very powerful and the same thing about you.

"And maybe it's because you are Americans speaking to Americans? And I'm an American? So that I can relate to that.

"And you're very good at relating this to people. Don't you think that that's an art that you developed?"

It was just a matter of doing for others what I'd want for myself, I responded. I'd want someone to make it tangible to me, like Bruce did when he took me in to work with that first patient, and I perceive that energy coming off of her and moving across her torso. I needed that, or else it was just a lot of words and hocus-pocus.

"I think they feel it, but you're just accelerating the power of it," he said. "It's like, if they do something like Tai Chi enough, they'll finally get it. But when you say it about the energy, they're able to look into the future and it helps them. Like they're able to say, 'Oh yeah.' Whereas if you didn't say anything, they might have felt something, but they wouldn't have been able to get that higher degree.

"That's what I think the value of a Qi Gong practitioner is. Just like a doctor who explains things, rather than saying, 'We're going to do these tests' and walks away. It's more powerful when you can look up and say, 'This is what it's doing.'

Sam suggested a future study that didn't offer explanation.

"But for now, you don't want to do that, because you don't want to get stuck on first base," he said.

Yes, I thought. Now was the time to hit home runs...

Sam asked about the design of the UC Davis Long COVID-Qi Gong study? I said the Principal Investigator conducted a waitlist control study, because it allowed for all the participants to get a shot at receiving the Qi Gong intervention, instead of just folks in the experimental group. In addition, there was one set of time points in which the waitlist group served as an internal control; that being, when the immediate group was receiving the Qi Gong treatments, and the waitlist group was still waiting their turn.

"Yeah, it's beautiful," Sam declared. "I didn't understand that before, but now, looking at it, I think it made your study more powerful.

"You know, your technique would probably be something that's great for rehab. For people once they've had surgery to be sure that they're going to come back and really recover to the extent of their capabilities. That's why I think you should go over there to Yale. They'll make you sweat, but I think they'll help you find the answer and it will be worth it in the long run.

"They're letting you into their home... To go to Yale. They're extending that.

"It's sad that the people who ran the UC Davis study didn't take it to the next step and try it with some other types of syndromes. Maybe people with malaria? Or people with autism? You wonder how it could improve their lives? Make them feel better?..."

Sam asked about the folks I'd trained in Qi Gong and whether they were positioned to keep my groups going when I left for Yale?

No, I admitted, sadly. Their lives were either dominated by matters pertaining to spouses, or work, or money.

He said that it reminded him about his ski school.

"I guess what I'm trying to say is, I understand your situation," he concluded. "It's hard for someone else to take it as far as you did.

"So, now you take it to Yale, and let's see if you can incorporate your stuff into someone's regular practice. They probably won't even call it, Qi Gong. They'll just call it their practice and mix it in a little bit with something they're doing in western medicine, but be able to feel their energy.

"It's sort of like religion. First, there was only one Christian church, now, there's a plethora of different denominations. They all kind of branched off, based on what the Lord's words were."

"But I think what you're doing is actually defining it," he concluded, "and you're making sure the essence of it is very powerful, and can be used in the best way, so that the results are even better…"

We talked about the first article from the Long COVID-Qi Gong study, in which we documented that those participants who didn't perceive Qi did not have improvements of their symptoms with the Qi Gong intervention, whereas those who did perceive Qi did experience improvements.

"How would you explain that?" he asked.

I thought it suggested someone had to tangibly experience the energy in order to derive benefit from it.

"But why didn't they experience it?" he asked. "What was the thing that blocked them? Was it because mentally they wanted it to fail? I have to think that that's probably it. They wanted to believe that it was hocus-pocus.

"I think that applies to Western medicine, too. You take someone to rehab, and the person just says, 'These damn stretches are bull', and doesn't get better.

"This isn't scientific, but it's my feeling that they should have felt it and derived healing. They are human beings, so it's sort of like biomechanics. If you work on somebody's bone structure, it works on everybody. When Stephen [bodyworker] works on somebody, and does his work, it works for everybody. There isn't someone that it doesn't work on. And it's the same thing with Qi Gong. The Qi is in everybody.

"So, I feel that it's a biomechanical issue. You have the fascia, the bones, the ligaments. You can call the energy the added thing. And when you do the alignment properly, you feel it. You can feel that tingling. You've got to have it in there. It's just got to be that some people aren't feeling it…"

I asked Sam why he thought I produced Qi from these points in my hands and arms that others could feel, whereas perhaps others did not?

"If it's just a matter of the energetic circulation of the body and that's something basic to all human beings, why doesn't everybody produce these points of energy?" I asked.

"I think there could be several reasons," he began, philosophically. "They always talk about that certain people have an aura, and some people have more of an aura than others. And what does it represent? I think that there are some people who have tangible energy and emit more Qi than others."

I recalled that my school friend Reuben said of me that an energy of joy surrounded me everywhere I went that he could literally see (until I got depressed in high school and lost it).

"And it doesn't affect their body temperature," he continued. "Because it has a buffering effect. You don't want to get the body too hot, so it releases from the body."

I initially thought it an astute observation; but then I remembered how it was when I was in medical school there were times I'd get frustrated and upset and become the "human torch" and suddenly "Flame on!", feeling heat coming through my skin, and wondered if it was because I didn't know how to modulate my Qi back then?

"And you have a greater sense of belief in it," Sam continued. "This also adds to that. It's very strong. And, also, I think you might channel into it easier than other people. Just like some athletes. Why do some people get it quicker when I train them in skiing? Some people take a long time to reach that level of achievement.

"So, I compare you with a good athlete," he declared. "You're just an athlete with external Qi Gong."

I'd always wanted to be an athlete, but being that my body was effectively broken from a young age, I never displayed any athletic ability.

Hence, to be regarded as an athlete of any kind was the fulfillment of the dream of a lifetime.

"And like a good football player or a basketball player when coached, they develop," he added. "And that's why I always wanted you to do Qi Gong on me. Because as long as you've done it on me, you're developing your skills better."

"So, I don't think anybody can just do it, but they're going to be some people who have better capabilities," he concluded. "But they also have to learn and practice to get better. They were just more ahead at the starting gate than others…"

"That's just my perspective and experience with athletes," Sam added. "And, now, don't you think things happen a little easier for you compared to when you first did it?"

Yes. When I taught students, I always wanted to leap into the most difficult experiences. When my students would describe a difficult energy disturbance that was just going around and around, I'd respond, "Yahoo, I can't wait to jump into that energy whirlpool."

"I think that you always enjoy doing it, but that you weren't doing it as cleanly as you could have," Sam commented. "And now you're fortunate to have a way to channel it quicker than most people."

It was more than that, though. Now, my energy experiences were so much more varied than they'd been before. When I started with Dr. Rind, it was just as a breeze that I experienced and only at my hands, which I followed across the room, millimeter to millimeter. Now, I perceived energy in so many other different ways, including "plugging in" at times, and being directed back to the person at others.

"You're actually controlling it," he asserted.

I didn't think it was a matter of control, because I felt I always tried to let Qi be in the "driver's seat."

"Then maybe 'managing it' is the best way to say it?" he responded. "All these 'variations' as you call them, you didn't have that in the beginning? You were just focused on one or two ways. And that's the point of development. You start with one thing, and you discover another.

"As I've developed in Tai Chi, I've discovered that it isn't just a strike, or a block, but it's a block and strike. And when you do that, I feel the power of both hands, so that the block becomes more powerful, and the strike. Because they're working together as a team. If I just throw this arm up, and then throw up the other one, then it just involves half the strength. But if I work with the two together, the strength is more than doubled. So, that's what I want to relate to you, because I have experienced it."

Still, more important for me than "control" or "managing" anything was what I did was purely patient-driven.

I thought that other Qi Gong Masters were no doubt controlling and managing it. I suppose that's when you really would use the term "external", because it came from outside of the person, and not from within. And I could imagine there might be a role when it was OK for a Qi Gong practitioner to direct his energy at an into a patient, like he was delivering medicine. But I suppose I treated myself like a therapist who was performing motivational interviewing and helping someone work through a traumatic condition him or herself.

"Like you're a guide?" Sam asked.

Yes, I said. I was looking to help a patient through what remained of the retained energy of trauma, so that they could resolve it themselves. I felt that the innate intelligence of the person contained the answers. And could provide those answers. And knew best how to answer the question of why that retained energy was still unresolved. And help the patient help him or herself to release that retained energy of trauma. I think the answer is in there and just needs to be coaxed out.

"I like that," Sam said. "I think that's probably the best way to do it. It's more harmonious…"

# CHAPTER FORTY

"When it comes to things like external Qi Gong that are borderline believable, it makes sense that people would say, 'This is hocus-pocus'," Sam asserted. "But I don't see it as hocus-pocus. I really don't. If someone called this hocus-pocus, then you might as well say that psychiatry or psychology is also hocus-pocus. Because it improves people's lives, too - though in a different way.

"I think psychiatry and psychology touch upon the personal aspect of this Qi Gong to really help people with their mental issues. But it's kind of limited, whereas your Qi Gong might not reach as high as it could, but I think it could improve people's lives and help them reach what they're capable of."

"So, you're fighting in a different type of realm of healing," he declared. "But you have to make it scientific. That's where I think Yale will help you. I have to tell you, Mike, you do not have an easy task. But I can't see anyone else more successful at it than you. It doesn't mean that you have to make it successful, but you're the best person who could possibly make it successful.

"I think it's pretty exciting," Sam said. "But it's interesting: Other people who go into things like this, they break up their marriages, they lose friends, but you've been keeping it all together."

It was hard for me to get too excited about it. Afterall, external Qi Gong was so unsteadied that there were no guarantees that I could offer about it.

Then, in that moment, I realized there was one guarantee that I could offer to my patients: I could tell them, "I guarantee you that I'm going to perform Qi Gong the same way that I performed it with the veteran who overcame neurologic deficits; and the elderly patient who overcame chronic pain and opioid dependence; and folks with long Covid who improved from the most common long Covid symptoms. That I can promise you. That much I can guarantee. The same way I worked with them, is the way I'm about to work with you. How you're going to respond, unfortunately, I don't know - That I can't guarantee."

"Right," Sam affirmed. "Exactly. That's all that people can ask for. You know, I'm just thinking about your future clients that you're going to have, and there's going to be so many varieties: There's gonna be some who believe in this stuff right off the bat. And others who say, 'I don't know? My wife told me to come and see you' and that type of person.

"But you have your credentials. And you have your self-experience. That counts so much.

"And then you've worked with a variety of different veterans and different types of people. All those things are going to increase and enhance your ability to help people.

"So, I don't think you can guarantee how you're going to help them. I mean, what do you say to them? 'I'm going to make you feel better'? No, you can't…"

# CHAPTER FORTY-ONE

It occurred to me that I hadn't offered to perform Qi Gong on Sam since we'd arrived at the hospital. In response, Sam said he was feeling weary and drained and would appreciate a Qi Gong treatment.

Performing external Qi Gong, I perceived energy at his solar plexus, which went outward and then strangely move my hand towards my Dantian, where it stayed for a while and it felt like it was because Sam needed nourishing energy from me to help him with literally his "seat of emotions", by extending to him what energy reserves I could offer.

Then, the directionality of the energy directed me back towards Sam's right hip, seemingly for the purpose of Chi emission, where my hand stayed for a while, and then move down his leg, and then up to his upper body, and then to his right hand, until ending at his right leg again.

I gazed up at the monitor and noticed that his heart rate had come down to the lowest point since he had been admitted to the hospital, at a healthy 68. Before that, it was usually hovering in the high 80s.

"I wonder if my heart rate goes up because my heart is trying to maintain the oxygen to my body?" he asked.

It made sense, though I thought it was mostly driven by the sympathetic nervous system, as it was my understanding that the heart is responsive to autonomic nervous system output.

As such, I felt concerned for how his heart was going to handle activity? Where his lungs were so compromised, his body was probably going to respond by speeding up his heart rate, and I was worried about how much his heart could take.

Sam asked me to scan him again for energy disturbances.

This time, I found energy at his solar plexus again, but instead of directing me upwards, it directed me downwards until it was solidly in my hand.

Sam indicated that that Qi Gong was helpful.

"The weariness is still there, but it isn't as bad," he said.

He said he thought most Tai Chi and Qi Gong being practices probably derived from older individuals suffering from debilitating, chronic and likely untreatable conditions, not unlike his.

"Most Tai Chi and Qi Gong masters are on the old side," Sam asserted. "And I think it's because when they're older, they feel a lot more in their bodies and can discern something that's a little bit painful. So, therefore, they are the ones who invented Qi Gong and perfected Tai Chi, even though they were debilitated and injured. In fact, I think the injuries helped them to perfect it even more, because when they do it correctly, it doesn't hurt so much."

Yes, I held that when Qi Gong practitioners were in the flow, when they were in a Qi Gong state, they are probably using their bodies in an optimal way, so that it doesn't 'hurt as much' (as he said) because the body has arrived at the goal of Qi Gong, which is to return the body to its optimal function; and once the body realizes that, then it will stop sending pain signals, because there's no longer any point to alerting the body that there is a problem, because the problem has been addressed to the extent that it can.

"Therefore, if that's correct, then there is an after-current to Qi Gong," Sam deduced. "Because by doing it correctly, the Qi flows easier, there's less stress, and it's not causing muscles to compensate. So, therefore, it tells this group of people, who are older in age and, like me, have kidney problems, stomach issues, bowel issues, 'You have everything', and that it's going to work to make their lives less painful and try to stabilize those medical issues and even cure those issues.

"And so, I think that's where Qi Gong really developed, and we are recipients of all these other people's dedicated efforts to make it healthier for themselves and others."

A product of their suffering, I thought. A gift to we who remain.

"That's why I say, for people to poo poo these things, that's really wrong. Because it comes from people who have been injured and had issues and perfected it to alleviate those pains and issues…"

# CHAPTER FORTY-TWO

Just then, our conversation was interrupted by two handsome, perfectly built, relatively young individuals (wearing masks and scrubs) entering the room and introducing themselves as coming from the Pulmonary Department.

"I'm the attending," said the woman. "Dr. Farkas is our fellow. He just wanted to ask some questions about your condition, if that's okay?"

Of course, I thought, excited. This is what we'd been waiting for.

The fellow began by asking Sam about environmental exposures? In response, we told them about his exposure to silicone sprays and rug fibers because of his ski business, asbestos that had been found in his home before being cleared, and tuberculosis in his childhood, which we understood were all associated with Interstitial Lung Disease.

In response, the two were casual and didn't take notes, and mostly nodded and offered comments like, 'That's interesting.'

When we informed them that Sam had plans for an echocardiogram tomorrow, the attending responded, "Yeah, I guess they can do that."

'I guess'? I thought. That seems an odd response.

Still, I felt hopeful, because they seemed so light about everything.

Then, in the most breezy of ways, the Pulmonary attending stepped in front of the fellow.

"I think our fellow is through asking questions," the pulmonology attending announced. "We reviewed your CT, and usually that's enough to make a diagnosis… No, we probably don't need to put you through a biopsy or anything invasive – The CT is usually adequate. It looks like you have something called PPFE. That's Pleuroparenchymal Fibroelastosis. And the reason that none of your previous treatments worked is because the lungs are so scarred that there's no way they can be made pliable.... No, antibiotics and steroids probably wouldn't do you any good. We were thinking about presenting your case at the Interstitial Lung Disease meeting on Wednesday at noon. We'll probably have some recommendations then. Hopefully you're at an age that you don't age out of lung transplant. That's the only treatment. Well, it was nice meeting you, sir..."

# CHAPTER FORTY-THREE

The Pulmonologists left the room as nonchalantly as they'd entered it. I stood stunned, feeling like I'd been hit by a truck. My breathing shallow, I stood statue-like, afraid to turn my head and face my friend and see the effect that their pronouncement had wrought on him.

Sam, meanwhile, went back to talking about Qi Gong.

"And the side benefit of Qi Gong is, it's preventive," he declared. "That's the key - Qi Gong and Tai Chi being preventive was not the focus in the beginning - It was to treat conditions. It wasn't just started to prevent problems. It was started to treat conditions. And this despite what anyone at the National VA says. Though, yes, it prevents medical conditions - That's why I would like my grandson to learn enough of it, so that maybe he'll live a longer, healthier life.

"I would like to do tai chi in my final days to alleviate some of these issues. That's why I'd rather be spending my time at home, instead of here.

"Because what am I doing here? I'm just waiting for tests. Whereas at home, I could be doing Tai Chi and Qi Gong."

Yes, I thought. Where these two "angels of death" from the Pulmonology Department had just essentially handed Sam a death sentence, what more was there to do here? In my experience, it came down to palliative care and being offered morphine.

"Yeah," he agreed, "whereas with Tai Chi and Qi Gong, you could flow and enhance your mobility a bit. And that's why I think your external Qi Gong is so important - Because it can start that process."

Yes, maybe give people some more death with dignity, instead of just a morphine-filled exit.

**"So, that's the way I would like to go," Sam concluded. "I just would prefer not to die with my eyes wide open..."**

# CHAPTER FORTY-FOUR

A nurse entered the room and announced that Sam's vital signs had remained relatively stable over the last hours, so she'd received orders to remove the telemetry devices.

They're done with him, I thought…

Working energetically with Sam after the pulmonologists gave him that death sentence, I followed the energy that extended from Sam with my left hand, until it connected with my first chakra, so that I could feel energy in my pelvic area.

"Ability to stand?" I thought. "Grounding?" Was he conferring that to me?

It wasn't until my crown chakra got activated that the energy left my hands, though it remained at my first chakra.

Sam commented that he felt like my hand was about a foot away from his eyes.

"I was thinking that you were right here," he said, indicating with his hand my expected location. "In my line of sight. But when I opened my eyes, I saw that you were over there across the room."

Yes, following the energy path, I was some 8 feet away.

"It made me think of something," he continued. "But first, tell me: Could you have your earphones on and your eyes closed and do this?"

Yes, I replied. Following the energy had nothing to do with hearing or seeing.

"So, as a test, what would happen if you were doing this with someone, and they quietly walked away, and went into another room?" he asked. "Would you be able to feel that there was a change? And the person wasn't there?

"Second, if the person was swapped with someone else, could you feel the change then? Not that I'm trying to trick you - Just as a scientific experiment. Could you feel that energy difference?

"I'm just curious if you could? If you couldn't, it doesn't mean anything. I'm just trying to understand how Qi works. It was just an interesting thing that I was thinking as I was sitting here - What happens if I wasn't here? And a new person entered? And you couldn't hear it? Would you perceive something different in the Chi? It was just a thought."

I don't know, and I don't think we'll have a good idea about any of this until we develop tools to be able to measure Chi. Before then, it's all just observation in this totally fertile ground for exploration.

"That's right," he responded. "You would have to measure it to know if you were truly detecting energy differences like that.

"But I don't think that means that this doesn't work; it just means that you're in tune with the first person so much that you were just carrying on. And maybe the Chi was maintained, because you were focused on that person? Who knows?"

Yes, it's a total mystery.

"Yes," he replied. "Just some thoughts as I was sitting here thinking – 'If I disappear, and Michael is still working on me, and I passed away, what would Mike be feeling? If I was gone?"

I thought that I would be connected with his energetic circulation, what remained essentially of his spirit.

Sam commented that he was feeling a lot of energy over his forehead, and indeed he was looking much more relaxed.

I commented that that was the space between his third eye and his crown chakra.

"That's right," he said. "It feels like it's buzzing."

Based on my understanding study of chakras, it was my understanding that function of the third Eye was to reconcile the conflict between our higher ideals (representative of the divine energy that we received at the crown chakra) and our basic survival instincts (which lay at the heart of our other chakras).

He commented that he also felt this kind of buzzing when he performed Tai Chi and Qi Gong.

"When you just relax and feel that tingling," he said. "I'm thinking that relaxing is what you're making me do, so that it enlightens my forehead and my brain - So that the energy is giving me feedback.

"I'm telling you this now, because I never told you this before, but I felt that before. So, it's nothing new. It's just I'm feeling it more. It's a nice feeling.

"It's like I told you in our last session, it felt like it had a calming effect, and I just feel light, like I'm not trying to trap something. There isn't that pressure; instead, it's like it's releasing the muscles."

I shared about my first experiences in Qi Gong with Master Chou, and how it was at the end of a practice, I'd experience all that clarity of thought; and I had no idea that I could enter such a state, because I thought the buzz in my brain was just natural and there was nothing abnormal or unusual about it. It was just a part of being. But it wasn't."

"That's how I feel!" Sam declared. "I didn't tell you that last night I was thinking that learning what I have about my condition here at Stanford, it gives me the opportunity to focus on my Qi Gong and see how far I can go with my Qi Gong? There's no other option to get better. There wasn't something to improve my condition, so now I can give it 100%. Versus before, there was always an alternative.

"So, now, I am free of alternatives. This is it. Either I perish or I go on. But now I can focus on Tai Chi and Qi Gong."

I agreed, though I wondered what kind of reception such a course of action would get from Sam's family?

"I'll cross that bridge when I get there," Sam said. "No, I've been thinking about this for a long time. Before, I didn't think I was going to die. But now, there is a twist, because now it's here."

It was late, and seeing that I thought tomorrow was probably going to be another long day, I got up to leave.

Sam lifted a tired arm and tapped me on the shoulder as I rose from the bed.

And making my way out of the ward, the feeling of energy in my first chakra persisted, so to leave me feeling like I had been gifted something that I would take with me into the rest of my days...

# CHAPTER FORTY-FIVE

After checking into a hotel, I called April and described the interaction with the pulmonologists.

"Very bad bedside manner," April commented. "How did Sam take it?"

In general, he's seemed less stunned than I was.

"Did they offer any comfort measures?" April asked. "Like in terms of how to make him comfortable?"

No, there were no discussions of that. Not even, "You might want to get your affairs in order. You might want to meet with our palliative care folks." Just, "It's maybe a lung transplant or you're dead."

"So, what did they say happened to Sam's lungs?" April asked.

They basically underwent some scarring process that was beyond repair, so that there was nothing that could be done about it. No treatments. Only transplant.

"And why did they get scarred?" April asked.

I didn't think we knew. Probably some immune reaction to either silicone that he was exposed to with his ski school, or asbestos that he was exposed to in his home, or the tuberculosis that he was exposed to as a child. It was either one of those things or a combination or who knows what his immune system just kept reacting against till his lungs were scared beyond repair.

And these guys weren't even going to look to evaluate any of those possibilities, because at this point, it didn't matter. The damage was done. There was no point in looking for a cause anymore. The train had already left the station. The crash had already occurred.

"Well, what I would do tomorrow before he gets discharged is to get accommodations for comfort care," she said. "Because unless he decides to go for transplant, which he didn't seem to be interested in, I guess this means hospice?"

"Because hospice is all about comfort care," she added, "and what can be offered to him to alleviate some of the suffering."

She broke off.

"I am so sorry that they had such awful bedside manner," she said. "You would never say that to anybody."

Yes, it felt like they were playing with us. Like a game of cat and mouse. Like they were toying with us - F'ing with us.

"Because they were asking those questions?" she asked.

Yes, they knew all along what Sam was dealing with.

If it was me in the physician role, I would have said to the patient, "Look, I want to hear what you've been through and learn as much about you as possible, but, in the end, there's something very serious that we have to talk about, because we reviewed your CT and there are some very serious decisions that we have to make here as we go forward." Not this 'easy breezy', "Well, it looks like you might have this PPFE, about the worst possible Interstitial lung condition that you can have, and you're only option is a lung transplant.

"And there's nothing that you can do to inflate your lungs?" April asked. "No medications will help you. You're just fucked."

That's what they indicated, I said.

"Did Sam seem interested at all in the lung transplant?" April asked.

No. Sam told me that he didn't want to spend what was left of his life preparing for a lung transplant, waiting and fighting for his place in line, sitting by the phone and waiting for the call that might never come, and then spending what was left of his life dealing with recovering from the procedure.

"I think I want to go home," he'd said. "And live the best way I can for the limited amount of time that I have left. And take care of my affairs, so that May is in the best possible position when I pass."

"Did they give him a prognosis or a timeframe at all?" April asked.

No, they seemed to indicate that they couldn't be sure when the next "dip" would occur. It could occur today, tomorrow, a week from now, a month, a year. They just didn't know. That was something that they would plan to discuss in the Thursday interstitial lung disease meeting over lunch, the said, and then plan on getting back to us about what the group thought of Sam's interesting case.

April released a sigh and cried.

"How was Sam before you left?" she asked.

On the one hand, he was cool; on the other, he was out of his mind.

He was sitting there in that bed, essentially staring into the great abyss. Death was upon him like never before in his life.

And on the one hand, he could let go. Because this is the way he always imagined that his life would end - Being pulled under into that great deep blue sea, just like when he was drowning.

I'd seen this before in people: When they've been hit with so much at one time that they just had to let it all go. That woman and Dr. Rind's office after being rear-ended again; Ethel facing her demise. A response to overwhelming stress, I suppose. You just can't fight anymore. The fight is over. And you know it.

"And the crazy thing is," April added, "if this was happening to anybody else, you would call Sam and talk to him about it..."

"Has May been involved at all?" April asked.

Yes, May and Sam's daughter, Sondra, came; however, both had to get back to managing things at home. Since then, Sam and I had been giving May brief summaries. But that stopped after receiving that death sentence, and Sam turned to me and said, "Mike, I know my wife and daughter are going to want me to fight to the end, and they're not going to understand my decision to let go."

I thought he was right, given I regarded May as a woman of action.

But Sam didn't want to fight to the end. He was accepting his fate. He was accepting things as they were. He was going into the great beyond.

"I really, really hope that they have some techniques, methods, drugs to alleviate his suffering," April said.

I thought it was just going to amount to the use of morphine.

"That's it?" she asked.

It was in my experience...

"So, you were not expecting this at all?" April asked.

No. I was looking for hearing things like, "We're going to rule out infection, and then we're going to start corticosteroids, and we're going to find a treatable source, and then, work to reverse all of this."

Because, from what I'd read, in general, interstitial lung disease has flareups, and then you give the person some steroids, to get over the flareup, and then you move on.

"The problem for Sam," April deduced, "is that he is at a stage where it's beyond that."

**Yes, I kept thinking about those pulmonologists and how matter of fact they were: "No, steroids won't help. No, antibiotics won't help. No, inhalers won't help."**

**"Well, what about giving them a try?" April asked, emphatically. "How would that hurt? Maybe they're wrong…"**

**She broke off.**

**"Oh my God, Mike," she exclaimed. "This is… Is there anything that you need? Or anything that I can do for you?"**

**I said that she had done plenty by sharing her thoughts, and now there was just getting some sleep and getting back to Sam in the morning...**

# CHAPTER FORTY-SIX

The following morning, I sat quietly with Sam in the hospital. While awaiting visits from his hospital doctors, Sam considered his attachments.

First was his grandson.

"I think my passing may put him at a disadvantage, but he'll be able to pick up things in other ways," he said. "He is bright, and he'll probably pick up things way before I did.

"And no one told me these things. They were things that I had to learn myself. Sometimes it's better if kids learn by themselves. I guess I'm resigned that he's going to do that. I think he's going to be A-OK. He's going to be fine."

"So, I know for me, I cannot let go of all my attachments," he continued. "The hardest one is May. But that can't be helped.

"The important thing is that you understand where I'm at with all this stuff. I have the feeling that they want to keep me here. But I think there's only so much we can do. It's diminishing returns. Unless they tell me that the corticosteroid treatment requires that I'm here, then it's fine, and I'm willing to do that. But, otherwise, I'm just looking at how I'm going to spend my time productively."

"Because, actually, it doesn't seem like there's a lot in it for me," he concluded. "I'm just walking another path in the forest. It's not that bad. It's just another path. So, I would not regret this…"

Sam commented about his first impression of me.

"I thought you looked like someone who was decent and smart," he said. "And who loved roller skating, like I do."

"And I think one of the coolest things when I watched you skate was your determination," he continued. "You made that face, and I thought, 'This guy is serious. Frickin A. Whatever he was doing, he was working on something. Because he was so intent. So focused.'"

And then, one night at the Rink, he reached out to me, and I told him that I treat this like rehab, and that my leg had been injured, and I was looking to reconcile the trauma and regain function in my leg.

"And then, you mentioned that you were a doctor," he said. "And then we went out to the Pho restaurant, and we made that a ritual - Which I looked forward to. I thought, 'This is really neat.' At the end of roller-skating, to sit down and cough in your face.

"And then I used to listen to you, talk about bioenergy. You didn't talk about Qi Gong; you were talking about bioenergy. Everything was bioenergy. Bioenergy.

"Then, all of a sudden, for some reason, I think you realized there was something even more interesting, and Bioenergy was just a sub-aspect of Qi Gong."

Yes, it because of him that I discovered that; the experience with him essentially took my Bioenergy and made it into external Qi Gong. That one day that worked on him changed everything. I was no longer performing bioenergy anymore; I was doing Qi Gong at its highest level.

So, who was Sam before we met at the skating rink? Like me, Sam had been someone who worked in science before being struck by injury. He'd risen from bench chemist to a Director of a Fortune 500 medical company. Working non-stop, he traveled the globe, helping start-up companies produce cutting edge bio-tech products to modernize health care worldwide.

Then, following a 13-hour flight from Asia, he experienced a 'snap' in his brain and found himself increasingly lethargic and unable to concentrate.

Seeking medical attention, Sam's doctors diagnosed him with a hypothalamic and pituitary disorder, with little hope of recovery. In response, Sam resigned his position and focused on preserving what remained of his health. Given the fatigue and lack of energy inherent in his condition, he looked to make the 'best use of self', with a focus on conserving energy through the efficient application of biomechanical principles. He applied this to his favorite hobbies – skiing and skating. This, in turn, ultimately stabilized his condition. As his health improved, he wondered if he could help others with chronic illness and established a ski school to teach others what he'd learned.

It was around this time that I accepted a position with the VA in Northern California. Given the proximity of my new position to the Sierra Mountains, I decided to take up skiing and skating myself.

Sam introduced himself at the skating rink, and we became fast friends, sharing our separate journeys through illness and healing as we skated and skied.

Close friends regarded Sam as like a kind of "life coach" to me, guiding and supporting my personal and professional goals, developing strategies to help me achieve them, and creating positive changes in my life.

But Sam was so much more. He was kind, selfless, and a source of beauty and inspiration. Being with him on the slopes was simply magical, like beholding a 'Ski Sensei', right out of the pages of Richard Bach's Illusions.

This gets me to the events that would forever change my trajectory in Qi Gong: One weekend, Sam confided that he was experiencing headaches so severe as to be incapacitating. This, in turn, got me thinking about that 'snap' in his brain that marked the beginning of his health problems.

Could these headaches be getting at the source of his affliction? I wondered. If so, could Bioenergy help?

I asked if I could attempt Bioenergy to try to help him? Sam agreed, and I performed Bioenergy. In response, Sam said the Bioenergy session had been helpful and provided some relief. But even as he thanked me for my efforts, I had the distinct impression that I could have done more and helped him better, and this feeling would not go away.

So, leaving Sam, I performed what turned out a long and convoluted Qi Gong self-practice, and, afterwards, I reached out to Sam and asked if I could work with him again?

This time, connecting with Sam energetically, something unusual happened: Not long after following the energy path of the energy disturbance coming from his head, I experienced an intense feeling of energy fill my hands.

Then, it was as though the Qi took hold of my movements and directed me back to Sam. It was as though the Universal Qi got inside me to direct my movements – like I was a puppet and the Universal Qi was pulling the internal strings. It wasn't me following the Qi anymore; it was the Universal Qi moving me.

This 'loss of volition' is characteristic of advanced Qi Gong performed at its highest level. I'd experienced it before, but never this intense and sustained, nor ever while working with a recipient.

There was no feeling of an external energy being involved; instead, it was like the Universal Qi had taken control of my brain, so to internally direct my muscles. Hence, the Universal Qi was guiding me 'from the inside', rather than my perceiving and following the Qi from the outside the way that I usually do and had taken control of my physical movements.

In this way I was directed back to Sam, and with my hands feeling charged with energy, they were guided to either side of his head, stopping within inches of making contact.

"It feels like I can feel all of the static electricity at my head coming from your hands," Sam said.

Indeed, I felt it, too. It was like energy was being directed from me to him.

"I'm feeling all of these pulsations," he continued. "And it feels like it's doing something."

Yes, this was Qi emission – what I'd been leery of and refused to perform for the last thirty years.

"I'm feeling the effects are all over my body," he continued. "All the way down to my legs."

Over time, the feeling of energy in my hands dissipated, signaling the end of the session.

"I really felt something happen with this," Sam declared. "The other time the feeling was subtle, but this time it was really definite. I really felt places in my body where they were healing as a result of this - Where I had healing - And the headache is gone."

I stood back stunned: It seemed that when I did that Qi Gong self-practice with the intent of being more helpful to Sam, the Universal Qi recognized that what my friend needed as Qi emission, and being that I was didn't understand how to perform Qi emission, it would essentially 'take me by the hand' and guide me through that process itself.

Hence, the Universal Qi or my innate intelligence or 'inner healer' or subconscious showed me how to perform Qi emission. It literally took volitional control of my body and movements to do that.

I want to make the point that it was never like I was 'possessed' or in a trance and didn't have control of my body; at any time, I could have resisted those movements. I hold that the Universal Qi was simply working at the level of my innate intelligence, so to guide me in performing Qi emission in a way that would help Sam and also help me.

And it was like the Universal Qi had to do this, because it recognized that, without its help (without it 'taking control' so to speak), I was never going to make that breakthrough on my own.

And what it did was show me that Qi emission could be performed in a way that honored all the tenets of my Bioenergy training; that is, I had sent 'healing energy' where Sam needed it, when he needed it, how he needed it and at the exact dose required, that was entirely recipient-driven, and without being forceful or involving any conscious effort. It was exactly the same as how I'd performed Bioenergy, except it involved a tangible and intense feeling of sending healing Qi.

As for Sam, the effects have been lasting, such that not only is he not troubled with the problems of headache, but the Qi emission helped him with his hypothalamic condition, as well.

"Ever since you worked on me, I don't have to focus on my pituitary or hypothalamus," he commented years later. "Before I always used to say, 'What's wrong with my hypothalamus? What's wrong with my pituitary?' But ever since you worked on it, I think it got better, so I don't have to think about it and I don't have to work on it, and it feels healed. I still take my testosterone, but the energy session helped out tremendously. And that's important, because I don't want a lot of medications – because I don't want the negative side effects associated with the medications to treat my pituitary or hypothalamus."

After that, my Qi Gong practice was forever changed and working with Sam got me over the proverbial 'hump' where performing external Qi Gong was concerned. It even happened with no effort or conscious thought. My thirty years of combined Bioenergy and Qi Gong practice had brought me to a place of performing external Qi Gong in gentlest, most recipient-driven way possible.

Being able to perform Qi emission solidified my place as an external Qi Gong practitioner. I had the full package now and had completed the circle of training I'd begun with Master Chou.

"All of a sudden your subject matter went from bioenergy to Qi Gong," Sam concluded. "It was pretty interesting stuff..."

# CHAPTER FORTY-SEVEN

Performing Qi Gong on Sam at the hospital, I started feeling energy around his chest, directing my hand upwards, then it directed my hand away from him, and as my crown chakra got activated, my left hand went towards me until it stayed stationary at about a foot from my solar plexus in which I felt a connection between my hand and solar plexus. It stayed this way for a while before I felt the energy directing my left hand back towards Sam, sending healing energy in his direction.

Sam said he was experiencing a beam of energy between my hand and his abdomen.

"It's not where my Dantian is," he said. "It's 3 inches below the diaphragm."

That's the solar plexus! I exclaimed.

"Yeah, and it was the first time I ever felt like there was a string attached to your hand," he said. "It was just a link. Like a beam. Just a light beam. A connection. No push or pull. It's like when you shine infrared flashlight against the wall. It's just like that. That beam. It doesn't pull. It doesn't push. It just exists. That's what I felt."

And this in the context of Sam having talked about the most important thing right now, being able to reduce his sympathetic nervous system activity, and bringing out more parasympathetic activity, so to stabilize his autonomic nervous system, instead of being in a fight or flight, stressed out state, which he contends is making things worse, especially for his breathing.

"And you know what, Mike, I'll tell you, just before we did this – when I was coming out of the bathroom – I felt like the end was near. It wasn't that I felt depressed. It was just a recognition that it could happen tonight or tomorrow. But at this point in the session, I don't have that feeling that tonight or tomorrow I'm going to die or pass away. I feel a little bit more optimistic and hopeful. Right now, all of a sudden, I feel lighter. It feels like right before I enter the roller rink, and I think, 'Maybe I can soar a little bit? See if I can impress myself and others?' That's what I feel like now. I feel lighter. I feel strong and agile. I feel relaxed. I feel upbeat compared to the way I felt downbeat when I stepped out of the bathroom and was like, 'I had to take this opportunity to talk to Mike, because I wouldn't be surprised if I passed away in the next two days.'

"Because I get this feeling on seeing all of this degradation. I say, 'Oh my goodness, something is going to happen. I'm going to slip away, if not tonight, maybe in a couple of days. Will I make it to the end of the week?'

"And I'm thinking clearer right now, and it feels hopeful. So, I feel really good right now. Just my body responding to you and your treatment. I feel more alert – Without being in sympathetic.

"Because when I stepped out of the bathroom, I was also feeling like I didn't want to be here and I just wanted to lay down. Now I feel like I want to go to home and get to my desk and do some bookkeeping, so that May and Sondra have a headstart on the income tax.

"And this is all in this very short time that you were waiting for me to come around the corner as I was coming out of the bathroom. I made that change in this very short time that I sat down and you did your Qi Gong.

"And I'm going to tell you," he concluded, "that's real. Because right now I feel upbeat..."

# CHAPTER FORTY-EIGHT

Just as Sam was about to undergo an Echocardiogram, an Asian man nonchalantly walked by the room. Sam called to him, excited.

"Stan!" he said. "Stanley!"

This was Sam's younger brother, Stan. Sam introduced me and asked me to describe his illness while he went for the echocardiogram.

After discussing Sam's illness, I asked Stan what it was like to grow up with Sam?

"With Sam, when he was growing up, he was just very, very smart," Stan began. "And my parents, along with my aunt and uncle, thought his education would be better up in northern California. So, after his junior year in Santa Maria high school, he went up north and started going to high school at Los Gatos.

"That was very devastating to me. Because, really, Sam was like a second dad.

"There were five of us. I have three sisters, one younger than me, and then two in between Sam and myself. So, once Sam left the house, I had three girls, three sisters, and it was all about majority rules, so it was really tough.

"My dad and Mom were farmers. Even before the war, my grandfather was a farmer. And all the sons worked in the field.

"So, when they came back after the war, and they started up farming again, and Santa Maria was the last stop for the Horishima brothers, farming. So, my dad never had time. He just worked. He was always busy. He was always working. Really 24 seven. All the time. So, when it came to sports and everything, Sam was the one who showed me how to ride a bike, play baseball, basketball, football. Everything with Sam. Sam was the one who taught me. So, in elementary school, when I joined a baseball team, instead of my dad, coming to watch the games, or coaching me, or teaching me how to catch, that was all Sam.

"And I don't have any grudges… I knew my dad worked. So, it's not like I was upset about it. But when I went to baseball practice, all the dads were out there, and then there was Sam - Who was out there helping out, hitting the ball to us, teaching us how to catch a grounder, how to catch a fly ball. Sam took the time to do things like that. How to catch a football. How to throw a football. That was Sam. You go out into the front yard, he taught me. Game of basketball, Sam taught me how to play basketball.

"And there was an age difference between us. But he always included me. With all his friends. His friends would come over, and they'd be playing basketball, and Sam included me. I got to play basketball with them.

"So, Sam was like a dad. My second dad. So, when he left, it was really devastating.

"Time went on, he stayed up north and went to college up there. So, I didn't have that mentor with me all the time. And I started screwing up in school. I call him on the phone, and he tried to get me on the right path again, but, of course, I was just a stubborn kid. In high school, all I did was just pass. Junior year, the counselor called me in and said, 'Hey, you're not graduating. You don't have enough credits.' And once my dad heard that, they sent me up north, thinking that would be better for me.

"And, of course, it was. So, I lived with my aunt, but Sam took me under his wing and said, 'Hey, look, you got to get your GED. I'll help you get your GED. I'll help you study. I'll do this and that. We'll get an apartment together. And I'll help you get your GED.'

"So, Sam was the one, along with my aunt, who was very concerned and didn't want me to be a bum. So did my parents, but Sam helped me out. By getting my GED and letting me live in an apartment with him, he saved my bacon."

"Sam was always there for me, but we always butted heads, too," he added. "Because Sam's a practical joker, and he likes to tease me, as a big brother should, but, man, we would get into these gnarly fights."

He roared with laughter.

"He would pick on me, tease me, and I would just get so upset with him," he continued. "He would get the point that he'd tease me so much that I'd get so mad, and I'd get physical with him.

"But there was a point of that I knew I had to back off. Because as patient as Sam was, he had a temper. But I just knew where to draw that line with Sam, because I was definitely afraid of going beyond that line, because he would kill me."

He laughed again.

"Sam was really a good role model. He always watched out for me. Always watched out for the family. He was the oldest, and maybe it was because that was what was expected of him. He was just a fantastic mentor and role model. And like I said, when he left, that was just very, very devastating for me."

There was an eight-year difference between he and Sam, and Stan was about eight years old when Sam left.

"I was still a kid," he said. "And he was always the one who I looked up to. He was very popular among his friends. He was very popular in high school. All his friends were sort of jocks. Sam was a wrestler, and he wrestled varsity. He was sort of like a stud.

"Even after I passed my GED… Well, when I moved up to Northern California with Sam, I was working three jobs, just to help out. And I realized, 'Hey, I don't want to live like this. I don't wanna be working three jobs.'

"So, when I decided to sign up to the police department, it was Sam and my uncle who helped put me through the Police Academy. They paid for it. Dad helped me out every way he could. At that time, Dad was very upset with me, because I didn't graduate, and he wanted me to take over the lawnmower shop because he didn't think I could make it. So, I had a lot to prove to my dad.

"So, with Sam and my uncle helping me out, paying tuition to get into the Academy, my food… They were the ones.

"Luckily, I passed the Academy, and three months later I was able to get hired. But I still had to pass probation and everything like that. And if I didn't have the encouragement from Sam, with him always being there, I don't know where I would be.

"So, I owe a lot to Sam…"

I shared that I found Sam essentially "otherworldly" in his enlightened approach towards people: Affirming. Supportive. Encouraging. Seeing the best in people. Wanting to be helpful. For me, he had been a tremendous source of support. As my wife said, whenever there was something that happened in my life, I always wanted to reach out to Sam to tell him about it (This to say nothing of all of the support he had given me with my Qi Gong endeavors).

I described how it was that I had something of an absentee father, who left us when I was five years old, and was usually so angry that he was completely incapable of teaching me anything; and Sam had been something of a second father to me, who would patiently teach me a lot of the practical things of life that my father didn't.

"Wow," Stan responded. "Wow. Sam is very fortunate to have you by his side like that. I just met you, but I don't know too many people who would be like that. I really appreciate it.

"But, yeah, you're right… Well, Sam and I, like I said, butt heads a lot, but I'll never forget everything that Sam's done for me. I would never be where I'm at if it wasn't for Sam.

"And I don't know if you know too much about my dad, and if Sam ever told you, but my dad suffered from quite a bit of PTSD. And as much as I respected him growing up, I grew up hating my dad, because he would snap. As I got older, even though I didn't agree with what he did, I understood that my dad suffered a lot, because of the wars, and it made him do certain things that weren't normal and weren't right."

Sam and Stan's father had the misfortune of having been visiting Japan at the time of Pearl Harbor. Despite being a naturally born citizen of the United States, he couldn't get back here and was ultimately drafted in the Japanese Imperially Army.

Then, after surviving the horrors of fighting for Japan during WWII, when Sam's father did return to this country, he was drafted to fight in Korea, served as sergeant, and saw some of the worst combat of the Korean War, wounded on multiple occasions, and witnessed the majority of his men get killed in battle.

"And he was definitely a provider," Stan continued. "And he would definitely do anything for all of us.

"And I was the only one who didn't go to college. One of my sisters chose not to, but she went to junior college. And my dad would have done anything to put me into college. Dad's goal was for me to become a doctor. But because I was such a screwup, that never happened.

"But my dad worked hard, and I got my work ethic because of my dad."

"I know my dad loved his kids, and my mom," he concluded, "but unfortunately, he did things in which he just lost control at certain times…"

"Sam and my dad and my mom," Stan continued. "I attribute everything to them.

"Sam, that's just how he was. He was the patriarch of the family. My dad and mom went through some hard times with the business, and Sam was there to help us.

"Unfortunately, we had employees who would embezzle and financially killed my parents. And if it wasn't for Sam and May... Well, financially, I wasn't in a position to help out... I got divorced. I was just always busy working instead of being with my family, so, unfortunately, that happened. Thank God I have a great relationship with my ex-wife and everything is about our kids.

"But Sam was always there. Even after my divorce, Sam was there. Sam was there for my parents. He would be there for any of my other sisters, if they needed him.

"So, I know where you're coming from when you say that Sam was there for moral support. He gave you the shirt off his back for anybody that he cared about.

"So, he saw something in you, Mike. He's a great friend, and when he treasures somebody, he'll do anything he could for them. I know you've known him for lots of years, so thank you..."

I asked Stan about Sam's near-drowning experience and how it affected Sam.

"You know what?" he began. "I'll tell you this: Sam changed a lot. And I can't pinpoint exactly the time. I don't know if it was when he was working for the pharmaceutical company? But something changed. And I don't know if it was because of the surfing? I don't know if he had a mental breakdown when he was working for the pharmaceutical company? But something happened. Because Sam changed. And I've always loved my brother. But because he changed, he always had these different opinions on everything. And it seemed like if we ever had a discussion about something, we clashed. And we never could agree on something.

"I knew Sam loved me, and I loved him. But I knew that I had to not get into certain conversations with him.

"It's sort of hard for me to be able to explain that. I wasn't there during the time of the surfing accident. But my cousin John was. And a good friend of ours was there. And the way that my cousin john, who was the same age as me, and we all grew up together, because we're cousins, and we're like brothers, too. But John just said, 'Stan, it was bad. The look on Sam's face. That's a near death experience for him.'

"So, I don't know if that didn't create issues, like medically for his lungs? Because if he was trying to survive, and it overworked his lungs?... Well, something happened, and I really can't explain it.

"I think I was working in Indio at the time, so that would have been 1984."

That happened to be the year of my life changing experience with Bubbles.

"So, by that time, I was working, and the only time we saw each other was on the holidays when we got the family together."

I asked about the change? In particular, whether it was a change for the better or the worse?

"For the worse," he responded.

He hesitated.

"But let me back up a minute," he said. "Like I said, growing up, Sam was always there for me. He's been there for me until this day. but something changed in him, and made it very difficult, even for my sisters, to have a conversation with him.

"When we would have talks with him, it was almost like he was antagonizing us. And if we had a different view on something, he would always make it sound like, 'No, you guys are wrong. I'm right.'

"It was just a weekend that we'd get together, but sometimes those weekends got hard, because we would get into discussions and then we would get mad at each other.

"I noticed that when I met his friends and other people, they had the image that he was there for them, like he was there for me when I was little. But when it came to family, especially his siblings, it was different. It was hard to have a normal conversation with him. Because whatever we would say, he would say, 'No, you should try this way.'

"It's hard for me to give examples, but it was to the point of being antagonizing all the time. So that it would get to the point where I would say, 'Hey, Sam, that's enough. We're done with this conversation now. Let's just move on.'"

"And I never saw it with the friends that he would introduce me to," he concluded. "But he still had the love for all of us..."

"I'm sorry that I don't know more about Sam's injury with nearly drowning," he concluded. "I'm sure that any near-death experience has effects. Just like for veterans suffering from PTSD.

"I know that when I retired, I realized I had my issues. But I missed the job. I miss the excitement. I missed the thrill of it. I love being put into different situations. Dealing with shootings. Dealing with when my partner got shot.

"People say, 'Oh my God, that's such a dangerous job.' But I never looked at it as being dangerous. I just love the excitement.

"And it might sound crazy, but I loved going into chaos."

**Probably like what his home life was like with a father suffering from PTSD after serving in two lethal wars.**

**"And I would coordinate things and say, 'Let's walk down to the location. We have a body down here.' I was able to make decisions on the fly. It was just exciting for me.**

**"Of course, I didn't like to see my partner get shot. Did he make the decision and do the right things? I only had to discharge my weapon once, but that was one too many times. I would have been happier if I never had to discharge my gun.**

**"But that's part of the job and you just deal with it and the situation that confronted me. And when I look back at certain things like that… I don't know. It was exciting. You try to make the right decisions and not put yourself in a compromising situation… I don't know. One day we'll have a drink, and I'll laugh a lot more with you..."**

# CHAPTER FORTY-NINE

Sam returned from the echocardiogram procedure, and I left the room, because I wanted him to have time alone with his brother.

I called April and confided that I'd been surprised that his brother showed up at the hospital, because I couldn't imagine that my brother would ever do that.

"But he drove up from LA?" April asked.

Yes. And he really wanted to spend time with me, and that he reserved a room in the same hotel where I was staying, so that he could take me out for dinner and we could talk.

And when I told him that I'd let go of the hotel room because I was expecting the medical team to discharge Sam this afternoon (and Stan was just going to be left with a room and a hotel bill and no me around), he let it go with just a laugh ("What's done is done," he'd said), whereas I would have been beating myself up to no end.

"What does Stan do?" April asked.

He's a former undercover detective, I said. Now, he takes care of his mother.

During the previous day, I'd listened as Sam spoke to his mother on the phone, never once complaining about his condition and just being reassuring to her, and left feeling like there was something about these two men – They had an aspect of maturity that was lacking in my brother and me.

My friend, Reuben, would say of my brother that he would act like "the man he pretends to be." It was the same thing with me. Somehow an aspect of maturity had passed us by. And that wasn't the case when it came to Sam and Stanley…

# CHAPTER FIFTY

Sam was, indeed, released from the hospital after the echocardiogram procedure. Driving Sam home, he said the members of his family had gathered at his home and he wanted me to help break the news to them about his condition.

April was also invited, so she came, too, and was moved to tears, later saying that she felt the way I discussed Sam's condition conveyed the seriousness of Sam's condition.

"One of the things I appreciated about your explanation about Sam's condition to his friends and family was giving them a visual and comparing the difference between the physiology of COPD and that of interstitial lung disease," April said.

I had told them that whereas COPD involve tissue destruction, so to create a confluence of the alveoli and reduce surface volume, whereas interstitial lung disease was a process that involved scarring everywhere, especially the subclassification that Sam had, which as well as scarring down the alveoli/air sacs so that they couldn't engage in air exchange, they were also scarring down the pleura, so that his lungs were literally being closed from the outside in, as well.

"And you told them that nothing could work for him as a result of that scarring," April said. "Not steroids. And how it was with COPD, you could give steroids, because there was a little bit of give, but for what Sam has, it doesn't. It won't. That visualization really conveyed and showed that there was some opening with COPD, but not for Sam."

Yes, everything was being scarred down everywhere, so that his lungs were being locked up and locked down.

Sam was in a place where he could just barely oxygenate his system. As long as he didn't exert himself and create a VQ mismatch, with the blood was running by the alveoli too fast to be oxygenated, he could maintain his current state; however, any exertion would put him in a place where he would not be able to adequately oxygenate his blood to provide for his body.

"So, in many ways, he's locked in," April commented. "He cannot tolerate exertion."

She said the description reminded her of an experience that occurred while she was working at the National Museum of American History.

"I worked on a very old, first-generation baseball that was made from natural latex," she began. "And a ball is supposed to be round and bouncy, but this one was desiccated and stiff. And that's the visuals that came into my mind about Sam's lungs…"

April said that Sam's homework was to be "chill" and commented that about how it was that Sam had essentially offered those instructions for his family.

"Sam told his family, 'You can't tell me how to fight this, because that will cause me stress, and that will cause me to leave this world even sooner'," April said. "Because I guess he really doesn't want them to push him. That he wanted to be in charge.

"So, it was very interesting the way he explained it, that when he's resting and unstressed, his lungs are able to get enough oxygen into his blood for him to feel normal-ish. But even slight activity or slight stress can push him under 90% oxygen and make him be sick.

"That wasn't something that he shared with his brothers as much, which I wish he had, because that might have made them help him more. He needs to be chilling out and letting other people do stuff around him. It's like he's telling them, 'If you want him around, he just needs to be chilling out

"But he's never been chill," she added. "And him being able to be with his wife and family depends on it.

"He has to just go with the flow and be like a reggae guy and just say, 'It doesn't matter.'"

Yeah, like learn from his brother Stanley, I thought.

But (truth be told) I was surprised that April had this take about Sam ("never been chill"), because I regarded Sam (as he would say) as "cool, calm and collected" all the time? I mean, compared to Sam, I was temperamental. I regarded Sam like Mr. Spock in comparison to me. So, what did that say of me if I thought Sam was so much more "chill" than I was?

**"You are able to let a lot of things go," April said. "When you give him advice, and he responds, 'No, I want to do things my way,' you usually say, 'OK, do it your way', because you're a friend…"**

**Then, the following morning, April woke up at 4AM, saying that it felt like there was some rearranging going on in her shoulder, and asked me to evaluate her energetically? She said that these internal rearrangements were helping her breathe more freely and were mostly centered around the trapezoid insertions at the spine.**

**"I feel like I can march in a parade now," she said.**

**It seemed to me that something had happened so to reach and remedy her shoulder problem at the "key lesion"; that being, the specific site of trauma that underlies all of the structural and/or functional impairments and compensatory restrictions throughout the body that resulted from that trauma.**

**Performing external Qi Gong with April, the energy move towards me in the direction of my left hip. Following the energy, it felt like I was dragging my left hip, and I remembered how it was that my mother would say of me that when I was an infant, I would drag my leg everywhere, and it was difficult for me to learn to walk.**

**As a result, I wonder that, just as April seem to be having a release at some very key lesion, if I wasn't being made aware of some key lesion in me? And whether we had not been imparted with a certain "gift" for our efforts to help Sam and his family?**

**Then, I noticed something else: While I'd been following the energy and performing external Qi Gong now, I wasn't perceiving the activation of my crown chakra? Indeed, it felt like it was back to what I was used to when I was working with Dr. Rind.**

**Why wouldn't I be connecting with a "higher source" now? Was it because the source had been imparted from Sam?**

**It was only near the end of the session that I felt a certain "tethering" between my crown chakra and the universal Chi...**

# CHAPTER FIFTY-ONE

Thursday, May 15, 2025

Returning to Sam's, I performed Qi Gong with him.

"When you were working on me, the right side of my head felt calm, but on the left side, I felt this vibrating," he said. "That was the first time I ever experienced anything like that."

I recalled that the day I had that major breakthrough and for the first time experienced Chi emission, it mostly involved Sam having a headache affecting that left side.

"Yeah, I remember that was painful," he said. "I couldn't bear it. It was just like a sharp needle or irritant there."

I'd been experiencing energy in my hands, but then it left my hands, and I felt energy at my crown chakra, though it was more on the left side, and had a tingly quality to it?

As for me, I'd been the victim of head trauma in my childhood, when a neighborhood boy threw a toy truck that struck me on the left side of my head. It was a problem for years and years, but hasn't bothered me so much at all that I could recall lately.

"Now, something is migrating over here," he said, indicating the left side.

Indeed, I was also experiencing something: the left side of my head, which I had towards Sam, was tingling, and my left hand was raised in a place right between our two heads, and I was experiencing a lot of energy in my hand?

And even more interesting, I was feeling energy at the back of my left hand? I don't think I've ever experienced energy at the back of my hand? All feeling for energy was essentially in the palms of my hands.

**"It feels like before I was in this high-level water at the left side of my head, and now it's pouring to the right side, "Sam continued. "Like the right side is building up and the left side is shrinking. So that, now, the energy on the left side is at a lower level at my head. Both sides are feeling equal and not as heavy as it felt when it was just on the left side. Kind of more distributed, and distributing things. And it feels like it's helping with my lungs. Like I feel this awareness in my chest.**

**"Now I'm feeling something in my legs and it's going all the way down to my feet. It's kind of like watching the sunset, and the shadow is getting longer and longer. And the shadow here is the energy moving all the way down. To my legs, to my feet , towards my toes."**

**Sam reported that he was feeling an ease in his heart following the Qi Gong treatment.**

**"It seems like everything moved out of my chest," he commented, "and went past it. It's like, I've been trying to use my mind to control everything… The rest of my body. And there might be a chance that we might optimize the situation for the lung transplant."**

**"That's what I want," he concluded. "To be stationary, because the pressure is going to be overbearing…"**

**Before departing, Sam thanked me for talking with the members of his family.**

**"You don't know how much that means to me," he said. "Because they're going to be the ones who help me, but I don't want them trying to help me and making it worse. So, having you to explain things helps so much."**

**Sam indicated for me to come back and give him a hug. When I did so, I couldn't help but accidentally blurred out, "See you tomorrow", even though I hadn't plans to do that.**

**"I would love that," Sam responded. "Although I wonder if that's a good use of your time?"**

**I couldn't think of a better use of it, I said...**

# CHAPTER FIFTY-TWO

Sam called and told me he'd got a call about his case review in the Stanford Interstitial Lung Disease conference.

"The gist is, they want me to go for a lung transplant," he said. "They said, 'Of course, you have to pass a battery of tests', and the one thing I had going for me was that I didn't require oxygen at this point…

In the meanwhile, Sam's wife found a well-known and regarded acupuncturist to treat Sam. I took the Amtrak train to Oakland, so I could accompany Sam to the acupuncture appointment.

The acupuncturist was an 80-year-old man who ran a very busy clinic, with people respectfully coming in and out. When it was Sam's turn, the acupuncturist repeated the spiel that I'd overheard him say to the last patient: That traditional Chinese medicine was about working with the body to get you better, and all healing came from the body, so that it was just his role to help the healing happen, and bragged about his part in bringing traditional Chinese medicine and acupuncture to the United States in the 1970's.

When Sam tried to described his many physical and mental symptoms, the acupuncturist was relatively patient. But when Sam finally got on the table, the acupuncturist was quick to insert about three needles in Sam's ear and instruct him to lay there for 45 minutes, before he would need to make room for the next patient.

Afterwards, Sam told me about what he experienced with the acupuncturist.

"When he took my pulse at those three points, it felt like your external Qi Gong," he said. "Let me put it that way, it felt like the two were very similar in that way. I know he was detecting a pulse, but it just felt like it was more than that. I wondered if he was projecting something at those three points? It felt like when I could feel your presence when you perform external Qi Gong and I go, 'Oh, it's like you're right there', even though sometimes you're not."

"The touch was really light," he continued. "It wasn't anything like pressure. Very light."

I said it sounded interesting, and I would have to learn more.

"Yes, I think it would be well worth your while," Sam responded. "Because it was like he was feeling the energy just like you do in the work you do. And it was a very soft, more direct contact. Because if I would've closed my eyes, I wouldn't have known if he was touching me that he wasn't touching me? It was more of like energy transfer. And that's something I think you should think about: but maybe there could be a touching component to your method? But it's a touching without a touching sort of thing. But it probably has to be right along some Meridian."

"And I think Steven [Sam's bodyworker] does that," he added. "He'll just tap me along my leg or arm, and although his is a little bit firmer, it has that essence of energy transfer."

"So, all those have a commonality," he concluded...

Sam asked what I thought of the acupuncturist? I said I appreciated the philosophy he espoused about traditional Chinese medicine being about enlisting the body to heal itself.

"Right, but that, in my opinion, is in all healing," Sam asserted. "It doesn't matter western or eastern. The western medicine just gives you more of an edge, so that your body can heal itself. Because your situation is so severe that you have to do something so that your body has a chance to be able to do something about it and not overwhelmed."

"It's like there are multiple army divisions fighting in the same battle," Sam analogized. "And one army division has much more heavy artillery; and when they take out the major artillery division, that gives the ground forces division a better chance to finish up that battle..."

# CHAPTER FIFTY-THREE

After the acupuncture appointment, Sam and May invited me to join them at their daughter's and son-in-law's home in Oakland.

Sam's daughter, Sondra, was a lovely young woman. His son-in-law, Jason, was self-assured and sturdy. They prepared a humble meal, and we all sat at the table together eating; however, the conversation was dominated by Sam describing his numerous symptoms, which I felt weighed heavily on everyone, and afterwards, I pulled Sam aside and told him that though I knew he was suffering and I couldn't imagine what he was going through, yet it was my feeling that he had to stay focused on what were his worst symptoms and not offer so many details to his family, especially as he had told his family that he wanted them to let him go through this process his way.

This left me feeling terrible, though. Afterall, I regarded Sam as the wise man who had guided my development over the last ten years. He had given me the input that had sharpened my mind and abilities. Indeed, working with him let me make that most important of leaps into chi emission...

"But he had to hear it," my spirit buddy, Steve, said when I recounted the experience later. "And it probably helped to hear it from you, who he respected. Sometimes it's important to say things like that. To wake somebody up. It sounds to me like he wasn't terribly aware of that - of how he alienates. So, I don't know that that's a bad thing that you did. He had to hear it from somebody he respected."

"He was telling his symptoms to people who are not qualified to interpret them or to analyze them," Steve continued. "He was telling them to the women in his life. He wasn't addressing it where it

**needed to be..."**

## CHAPTER FIFTY-FOUR

As well as being worried about Sam, I was also worried about me – because Sam was all I was thinking about, and I was having a hard time focusing on anything else.

Steve thought I was spending too much time "externalizing."

"One thing that you might consider is that you can still be very concerned about Sam," he began, "but Sam is external to what you are actually working on and need to be doing professionally right now.

"As it is, it's this whole thing of external circumstances, and how they can so influence you to the point that you can no longer focus on what you need to be doing internally and what energy you need to be working with internally.

"Certainly, you can be aware of the external circumstances, but when you allow them to take your entire focus, take everything of you, then you are totally depleting the energy and externalizing all of the energy that you need to use in building up what you need for yourself right now. which is all this focus on where you're going professionally. Focusing on the paper that you need to write right now. The substance of what you're bringing to Yale, so that they can put it into the form that it needs to be in.

"But by focusing completely on Sam, you're externalizing all of your own energy and it's taking it away from where your energies need to be.

"And part of this is because you do care so much about other people. I get that. You really do. But sometimes it is not selfish to say, 'It's time on where my energy really needs to be.' And your energies need not to be externally, focused on others right now. They need to be focused on your process. And not only in a professional

**type of way, but in a way that you're focusing internally on the strength that you have. And too, too much of that right now is being depleted externally on Sam."**

**April, however, felt differently.**

**"I see where Sam is such an important person to Mike," she said. "I see whenever Mike is struggling with something or wants to share something, Sam is like the first person he talks to. It's like Sam is a chosen, very close brother basically. He is a family member."**

**"But it makes me think about one of Mike's biggest gripes when it comes to his dad," she continued. "That when he was in college and he met Bubbles, and his dad was like, 'You need to concentrate on your studies. That's more important than a girl. You'll find girls some other time, but right now, you should be focusing on your studies.' And later on, Mike wanted to build a life with her, but it was too late, so that's part of the regret.**

**"But I would trust Mike to know what he needs. I know that some people can get into an eddy and focus on others, and not take care of their needs. But I also think that it's way early for that."**

**"I mean, it's only been a week," she concluded, "and I try to trust his judgment…"**

# CHAPTER FIFTY-FIVE

Talking with my therapist about Sam, she asked what I really thought about his condition? I said I thought Sam was a ticking time bomb, because one of these days he's going to get that upper respiratory infection, and then he wasn't going to be able to fight it, and that was going to be that.

None of the normal systems that other people rely on were working in his lungs, I said. There was too much scarring for things to be cleared out, or oxygen exchanged, or for him to be able to use his muscles to breathe.

The scenario that I envisioned in the near future was him winding up with a respiratory infection that landed him in the hospital, where he would die.

He simply doesn't have the reserves to fight off anything, I declared.

She asked if it felt like a "gut punch"? I said the gut punch was those pulmonologists delivering the equivalent of a death sentence that took all hope away.

"If you felt like you've been delivered a gut punch, you wonder how Sam felt?" she said.

I think he felt the same, though, at the same time, he was so kind and talked about his hopes for me to advance my work. It was quite an extraordinary evening in which I really felt connected with him.

So, it was funny to be back at work and effectively disconnected from him. It didn't feel right.

"You're like brothers," she said. "Such a good friend. I'm so sorry…"

I said I was afraid that Sam wasn't operating from a prepared place. I felt he was not prepared for all the possible eventualities. Because he was walking on a tight rope, and he could blown off with the slightest, little breeze at any moment, and then, unfortunately, my friend could be gone.

"That's a shock," Barbara said. "So, you don't see much of a chance of him getting the lung transplant?"

No, I didn't think he was going to make it. I didn't think he had enough reserve. I would be surprised.

"It's a lot to take in," she responded. "Cope with. Process…"

# CHAPTER FIFTY-SIX

Calling Sam, we talked about my plans to go to Yale. For a number of reasons, I didn't want to rush leaving here, but wondered if I was being too relaxed about the whole thing?

"I like that strategy," Sam said. "And that is a strategy, because you at an age where you can do that. If you were younger, I would say that you should take the position right away. 'Jump on it.' But now, I think you can be more mellow. Because you've got a lot of experience behind you already. When you're young, you need to be gathering experience. So, you have to jump on things. Now, I think you can be a little bit more calm about things. Is there a risk with the calm approach? Yes, but I think that you have a grasp on it."

I confided that there were those in the Qi Gong research world who wanted me to start the Yale position right away.

"Do you think they have ulterior motives?" Sam asked.

I knew they did: They had wanted me to help them set up a Qi Gong conference at Yale, because they said that would attract more people than a conference at a smaller college.

"It sounds like their advice could be on the selfish side," Sam responded "So, I wouldn't put a lot of weight on someone with advice who could take their interest over you.

"I think you have things well at hand. I think whatever comes up, you will come up with the most reasonable answer. I think you've been through the gauntlet. You have experience, you have things to back you up in your thoughts and in your ideas.

"To be honest with you, Mike, I think you're in a very wonderful position. You are in a position in which you can call most of the shots yourself. Maybe not everything, but a heck of a lot more than most people given your breath of experience."

Yes, I told him that I thought if I went now, my head wouldn't be in the right place, because it would be back here, thinking about him and my father and finishing off the paper about the long Covid project. I think I'm better off as a person by waiting until October.

"I have to say you have to go with your gut," he responded. "Because you're right, if your head's not in the right place right now, and you know that your head will be really solid later, then I think you're doing the right thing.

"I will say this, though: Your dad is not going to get better. And if he is still around in October, you're still going to have that pressure. The same with me: If things get delayed and they can't find an organ that's right for me, it could last through that time. So, things might not change that much. But one thing that will is that you will be changing and evolving, and you may be more prepared.

"And maybe you can get a few things started without this having to go physically go there? So, I would start laying down some foundations for your work from afar. Tell them that you're serious about going to Yale. And that you want to get things rolling, such a grease the skids for your landing. And that way you might find something that satisfies everybody a little bit. And a little bit may be enough. And I think it might make you feel good, too - That you're not asserting yourself on them, and you're prepping yourself for running really fast. You're not just coming out of the gates - You've already got some traction."

But could I do those things? It seemed to me that I disappointed these folks a year ago by not coming. How could I reassure them this time that I was coming, and I wasn't just a boy who cried wolf? Should I tell them what a difficult year of the suspend? That we became homeless because I felt like things weren't quite right, so I held things up? Would that help reassure them that this time I wasn't pulling out?

"Well, look, you can tell them, 'I got a temporary living arrangement right now, and I'm not looking for any place here. Indeed, I'm trying to get the feel for where I could be living in New Haven.' That's why I think it's nice to talk with these people on a constant basis. Because that way, you're always moving things a little bit forward. I think constant communication is going to reassure them. I think the things you're talking about would be valid if you weren't doing anything. but if you do some little things like what we're talking about, then I think it will allow them to think that we're moving ahead here, even though you're not physically there yet."

"It's sort of like a chess game," he concluded, "and you're moving some pawns..."

"So, do what you feel is right," Sam continued. "And in the meantime, with your dad and stuff, you know you're going to be going over to the East Coast and your dad is probably going to still be alive, and his condition might be sinking a bit more, And you can sort of prepare yourself there, about how you're going to continue your communications with him, and what you need to leave for when you're not around.

"And make sure your father has some good peace. So, as he's moving through the phases, there are ways to keep in communication even from a long way and that makes him feel good.

"And when it comes to me… Mike, you don't have to worry. I have so much support from family and friends. I'm a very fortunate person.

"I know you worry, because you're a friend, and so I'm not going to say, 'Don't worry.' But when I'm trying to say is, 'Worry less.' Because I have a lot of support. And I will call upon you and your expertise every once in a while, so just help me in those little ways. That would be fantastic, like you've helped me this much.

"This is the neat thing, Mike - You shouldn't be spending a lot of time on what needs to proceed for me. Because you're a doctor, it will come naturally. You'll hear about something and then you'll say, 'Oh, yeah, Sam you should do this.' That's all I expect. In fact, that would be so valuable, because it's coming from an expert and from you. You don't have to worry or spend a lot of time. Because the help you would be giving me will be spontaneous and very targeted and specific. And it shouldn't be a burden on you.

"So, worry less is what I'm saying. Because your help will come spontaneously and naturally and freely. So, it won't be a burden on you.

"Because, Mike, you're a Doctor, who has many years of experience. So, all I need to know is your thoughts when I have certain issues, and you'll come up with the answer.

"So, don't spend your time worrying about me. Spend your time worrying about your program. That's more important. And I have the feeling that as your program improves, you're going to find ways to help me better. I expect to improve because your program has improved…"

I told Sam that tomorrow night, Wednesday, is when my Post-Study Long COVID-Qi Gong group meets.

"You need to get as much out of those meetings as you can," he said. "Because you're going to take that knowledge and experience with you to the East Coast."

I asked if he'd be inclined to meet the group, where I consider him the most important person in me advancing to becoming a full Qi Gong practitioner with the ability for Qi emission?

"That's a heavy honor you placed on me," he said. "Let's play it by ear. Give me a call when you're leaving to go over there. If you think that's a great value, I'll see if I can make it. I don't know how I'm feeling day today? I'd like to be feeling like I am today on tomorrow. But we'll see?"

I asked if I could bring the group to him at his home, so he didn't have to travel to the medical center?

"I think it would be better to be in their setting," he said.

But I didn't want him to exert himself by traveling to the medical center.

"Yeah, but I don't think May would appreciate a lot of people coming over who she doesn't know," he countered.

I told him that I would call then.

"Yes, let's see how I feel then," he responded. "Maybe what you could do is FaceTime me?... Let me know as the day progresses. Maybe after your work? Sometime after five and around six maybe we'll talk?"

"So good talking with you," he concluded. "Everything you do, I appreciate. OK, I better get some rest..."

# CHAPTER FIFTY-SEVEN

Wednesday, May 21, 2025

Ruth and Rosa arrived late to the Post-Study Long COVID-Qi Gong group, saying they got caught in the traffic jam (probably an accident) on the way to the medical center.

I called Sam and introduced him, saying that he was my best friend and confidant here, and reminding the group about the experience with Sam that confirmed me as a Qi Gong practitioner, capable of performing Qi emission.

Then, Sam introduced himself to the group and described his condition, speaking in his usual metaphors.

"I started from a mountain top," he began, "in which I had a pretty good view, and this year, I fell from that mountain top, and just so happened to land on a ledge. But that ledge is much farther below where I started. However, even when you're on a ledge, you're still on the mountain, and there are some good views even from here. But I keep slipping a little bit more and going down and landing on another ledge. and I'm trying to enjoy that view, as well. And I think the external Qi Gong helps me enjoy that view at that ledge a little bit more. And makes life more enjoyable. And I'm not going to say that Qi Gong could cure it, but I think Qi Gong could reverse some of it and allow you to stay on that ledge a little longer…"

Sam described input he'd received from the medical community to treat his condition.

"Like the doctors are telling me that I should take the anti-fibrotic because it may give me a little aid," he said. "And a little aid for me is a big aid. And that's just like external Qi Gong could be that little aid that amplifies for me as a source of help, allowing me to enjoy life a little longer at a nicer place."

Sam talked about the benefit of his nebulizer treatments.

"They don't change the scarring, but they help make it so that the things that are blocking my lungs get out of the way. It makes my condition so that other things don't add to the problem," he said. "And Mike understands the mechanisms of my disease and the anatomy of the lungs, so I think that makes his Qi Gong more focused…"

Then, Sam talked about the theoretical origin of Qi Gong.

"When people are healthy with normally functioning limbs and organs, most of the time they can't feel the effect of Qi Gong," he began. "Because there's nothing wrong to be fixed. Whereas when you have some active disease process or chronic painful condition, then it does create disturbances within the body that facilitates a certain sensitivity to the perceived effects of interacting with the energetic circulation."

Sam had been exposed to tuberculosis at an early age that produced significant scarring in his lungs and possibly progressed to his terminal illness.

"And you have to imagine that in China and probably any place around the world, TB ('consumption') is a common disease. So, you had people with this illness (probably similar to what I have now) for thousands of years, and they had to deal with it and find ways to make their lives go on. Because they couldn't just rush to an emergency ward back then. They still had to plow the fields, feed their families, do whatever. So, they had to find ways that would just get them through the day, even under harsh environmental situations.

"And, so, they had to figure out more ways. But these folks were more sensitive to their environment and to their internal processes. So, they were able to feel things, and I think that laid the ground back then to find ways that would ease them. And things like external Qi Gong with something that provided relief. And that's where it developed.

"Because I don't think that things like that developed when people said, 'You know, I think it would be fun to do something I call Qi Gong.' That's not the way it happens. There has to be a need to develop something, whether that's infection or injuries, which were more common back then. And the forces against trying to survive one day and find food and find shelter and everything else like that, demanded ways to figure out 'on the run', so to speak – How to feel better, so that they could accomplish a day's work that would allow them to survive."

Yes, Qi Gong was their medicine, I thought.

"I can't prove it," he concluded. "But that's what I feel. And the help that it gives me ... Well, even a little bit is a lot. Because every breath I take is a struggle and it has been progressing to this point..."

As Sam was speaking, I was actually having an interesting Qi Gong experience: Connecting with the energy within myself and everywhere around me, it was directing my axial skeleton move around and around my pelvic bowl.

Later, I had the rare experience of feeling like a "well-oiled and integrated machine."

I wonder if the revolutions of my axial skeleton around my pelvic bowl didn't free up something? I felt more free in the lateral aspect of my left hip and wondered that that didn't play a significant role in my ability to be grounded and walk is an integrated unit.

Ruth would comment later that she thought Sam had an "activating" effect on me...

Next, we performed the self-practice. As I led the group through the self-practice, Sam shared that he was feeling energetically.

"It's just like when I perform Tai Chi or Qi Gong," he said. "I can feel the pressure of the ball."

Sam indicated that he was not experiencing energy at his crown chakra, and, instead, was perceiving a distinct directionality of the energy in his hands.

"My hands are now separated, two feet apart," he said. "It feels like I'm holding a very solid ball between my hands. My hands are pulsating and want to move in and out. They're not rising. It's definitely very strong. It wants to keep my hands there. If I would try to collapse it, I would have to put some force into it. If I want to separate them, I have to put some force into it, as well. But where it's at and pulsating, it feels very comfortable to me there. It's like they're just suspended."

"I'm very calm," he continued. "As you can see, I'm not coughing now. It's calming me. It feels very comfortable. There's no strain. It's like my arms are floating there and I can hold it and feel like, 'Wow, it's just staying there.'"

I suggested he be with the energetic circulation for a while. It happened that he was not feeling the activation of his crown chakra, and this didn't surprise me, because when we were in the hospital, and I was working with him, for whatever reason, for the first time in years, I was not experiencing the activation of my crown chakra as I followed his energy disturbances? Otherwise, since the first day that I worked with participants in the Long Covid-Qi Gong Study, I experienced the activation of my crown chakra, as though to indicate that I needed some external source to help me to help these long Covid patients; whereas I didn't seem to require that with Sam?

"I'm starting to feel everything dissipate now," Sam commented, "and my hands go back to normal. Just relaxed, and now my hands are resting on the table. I'm not feeling any pulsating or something keeping my arms up. But it is relaxing. I feel very relaxed. And my mind feels uncluttered…"

Rosa commented that Sam had a relaxing voice.

"I could just meditate listening to you talk, Sam," she said. "Very, very lovely meditative voice."

"That's nice of you to say," Sam responded. "I feel my voice is very tired and a little bit strained from my standpoint."

Just then, Sam entered a fit of coughing.

"Mike, I think I'm going to have to excuse myself and get something to drink," he said.

With that, he thanked everyone and got off.

Rosa made the point that Sam said he trusted me, and she felt the same way.

"From the moment I came into the room [for the Long COVID-Qi Gong study] and you introduced yourself, I felt like, 'I can trust this person'," she said. "And I don't think I would have been open to Qi Gong or the benefits of Qi Gong or any of that if I didn't feel that trust where you were concerned. And Sam talked about having that feeling about you, and I think it's really important..."

## CHAPTER FIFTY-EIGHT

Thursday, May 22, 2025

The morning after virtually attending the Post-Study Long COVID-Qi Gong group, Sam sent me the following text:

*The session with you and group was very relaxing and powerful for me. The energy in my hands felt stronger than I have felt than any time in the past holding the chi ball. Maybe that had something to do with helping good sleep, healing and good feeling this morning. Thank you!*

Later, though, Sam called and described feelings of pain in his chest that he thought was associated with his near-drowning episode and the vicious cycle of shortness of breath and anxiety that it manifested.

"Trying to breathe into my lungs and open my chest, I feel a strain," he began. "It's just not getting oxygen, and it's the same feeling like when I was drowning. Like when you're out in the ocean, and you're trying to breathe and looking out, there was no land in sight, and you're out there and you're just going, 'Oh, man, it's almost like it's hopeless. I don't know how long I can keep this up. I'm exhausted. My muscles are sore. I'm taking in all this water. And I'm fatiguing. And I'm losing my sight and it's cold. And I'm trying to not take in the water, and I'm straining to breathe.' And every once in a while, I get that feeling, because I feel like I'm trying to breathe, and it's not happening, and it feels like someone's hitting you, and I'm just struggling, and it doesn't feel manageable..."

His comments reminded me of what Ruth said had said about him after he got off the call last night - That, listening to him, it sounded like he was "drowning"…

"I think more than a panic type of pain, I'm having a struggling pain," he continued. "That's the word I'm looking for. It's more of a struggling pain. And I think it's psychological, too. My mind moves me into more of a panic type of situation."

I recalled my experience with COVID-19 and the tremendous anxiety associated with feelings of shortness of breath.

"Oh, yeah, that's part of it," he agreed. "The shortness of breath can set that off. Whatever is going on it's a struggling pain. Like you're trying to stretch something, but it's not stretchable."

Like everywhere in his lungs, I thought, which were now entirely scarred over – and beyond them.

"It just seems very restrictive," he said. "It's like you think that something should be movable, but it's not. And you keep pressing against it, and you think, 'I know I can move it', so you keep pressing, and you feel the pressure, but it's not moving. It's that kind of pain. And when I'm having my anxiety attacks, I can't breathe. And you're trying and struggling, and your lungs won't work. And you're just pushing it and pushing it, and it just won't open…"

I asked if these feelings and experiences were causing Sam to relive his near drowning experience?

"Sure," he said. "So, I'm just trying to figure out which one is psychological and which one is physical? And I'm fighting against the scarring and contractures that won't stretch, and relax and take in oxygen."

"So, there are two things here," he concluded. "One that I'm creating mentally, and then there's the other one that's physical, such that it's physically impossible to breathe. And as I approach that stage, I'm just wondering, 'Is there a way that I can manage that pain in a safe manner?'…"

I confided that I didn't want him to suffer, and I had been wondering about the use of opioids to treat his pain and cough and anxiety and shortness of breath? The conundrum is, Opioids depress the respiratory centers, so they could possibly hasten his passing.

"Right," he said. "I wasn't thinking about that right now. I was just thinking if things got worse. That's all."

I shared how it was that during the pandemic, I kept a written statement with me at all times, describing my near-drowning experience, which left me with problems of air hunger and severe anxiety associated with shortness of breath, and saying if I had Covid and it got to my lungs, so I required intubation, then I wanted to be placed on heavy doses of morphine and kept on morphine. Because, for me, every second that I have that anxiety feels like a lifetime, and I'd rather be kept in morphine-induced dreamland, even if that meant dying.

"Yes, but for me, I'm just thinking, 'What is the gentlest thing this way?' Because I know that I'll probably need more and more pain medicine, but at the beginning, I don't think it's going to be that much. I just don't want to have too much at the beginning. I just want to, how would you say, soften the edges. Because I'd like to be as [mentally] clear as possible."

"So," he continued, "those are the things that are on my mind as I'm getting more of these struggling pains leading to anxiety. I think it all comes down to pain management, because I would like to be as lucid as possible, but the anxiety and pain…"

He broke off.

"So, I thought I'd let you know my wishes," he concluded…

## CHAPTER FIFTY-NINE

Sam indicated he had friends coming from his hometown in Santa Maria.

"But, as always, you're more than welcome to join us," he said. "It's always nice, and I can introduce you to them..."

Ending the call, I took a deep breath.

I didn't want to be lucid, I thought, considering my friend's situation. Rather than pain and anxiety, I wanted to be out, and I rather wanted that for my friend, as well.

Then, I got a call from my brother and related my conversation with Sam about how utilizing opioid medications could hasten his death, versus lung transplant, which invited a life full of difficulties.

"Because if it was me in his situation," I said, "I'd just tell them to give me the morphine and get it over with."

I wouldn't be willing to live the way he was, I said. I didn't want the added experience. I just wanted to check out of this life and move onto the next one - This despite supposedly being a change agent and having such a mission to accomplish in this world.

"Life is a one-time deal," my brother responded. "So, if there's opportunities to get another year or two years or however many, sometimes people are willing to accept pain for the time.

"While others say, 'You know what? The time could be better spent slowly relieving the pain and riding off into the sunset'..."

Then, out of the blue, I got a call from my "long-lost love", Bubbles, who wanted to comfort me after sharing what's happening with Sam.

"What you're going through is just horrible," she began. "So horrible it makes my heart ache, just thinking about what you're going through. I just know that you've mentioned Sam all these years and he's been such as a source of support for you. I just feel so bad for you."

Yes, this mentor of 10 years was so extraordinary - Even as he was confronted with his mortality and offered the worst news of his life, he was still conveying all these sentiments that were so uplifting to my heart.

"That's what my mom was like the whole time that we were sitting there being all sad and crying," he said. "She was still taking care of us. What a wonderful man he is. In what ways was he your mentor?"

He always captured the essence of whatever I was trying to do. He would give great advice, full of allegories and metaphors.

I shared about how it was that he referred to me as an athlete of the energetic circulation and, given I'd lived in the shadow of my incredibly gifted athletic brother (while I'd dragged a twisted, broken body everywhere), his comment made my lifetime.

"That's definitely a good way to put it," she responded. "Because you're an athlete in your brain."

She laughed.

"That's what I think of you," she continued. "I think you're so in touch with your whole self and able to understand yourself. Because you can't help people if you can't understand yourself. With me, I get caught up in myself, with my problems, my ideas, my goals, whatever. And then I have to be rescued from myself, because I take everything to some sort of extreme, until somebody says, 'You know, that's just not going to work out the way you're approaching that.' But you just seem to naturally have that ability of knowing yourself. Introspection. That's the way I've always thought of you."

But in this way, too, compared with Sam, I was the merest of amateurs...

In response to telling Bubbles about Sam's recent experience in the Qi Gong group, she was encouraging.

"It sounds like you were able to help him," she said.

I replied that felt deeply for Sam's breathing difficulties, because I had my own residual PTSD from my near-drowning experience. Indeed, to this day, whenever I go into a sauna or sweat lodge or had difficulties breathing when I had Covid, I go into a panic, so that every minute feels like a lifetime of horror.

Then, Bubbles offered an insight that I hadn't considered before.

**"That's the opposite of what you do with your energy," she commented. "It may help him to relax, so that his airways can open, instead of…"**

**'The opposite of what I do with my energy'? I thought, pondering her comment. As though my Qi Gong self were my alter ego?...**

**"How was Sam your mentor?" Bubbles asked. "Is Sam a Qi Gong practitioner or Qi Gong master or does he just support what you do?"**

**I said that Sam had taken up Qi Gong of late, but over the years, he'd mainly been a source of support and talked about the experience of chi emission with Sam, and how it was that before that, Qi emission just didn't feel right to me, and I wasn't willing to do it.**

***Not long after following the energy path of the energy disturbance coming from his head, I experienced an intense feeling of energy fill my hands.***

***Then, it was as though the Qi took hold of my movements and directed me back to Sam. It was as though the Universal Qi got inside me to direct my movements – like I was a puppet and the Universal Qi was pulling the internal strings. It wasn't me following the Qi anymore; it was the Universal Qi moving me.***

***This 'loss of volition' is characteristic of advanced Qi Gong performed at its highest level. I'd experienced it before, but never this intense and sustained, nor ever while working with a recipient.***

***There was no feeling of an external energy being involved; instead, it was like the Universal Qi had taken control of my brain, so to internally direct my muscles. Hence, the Universal Qi was guiding me 'from the inside', rather than my perceiving and following the Qi from the outside the way that I usually do, and had taken control of my physical movements.***

***In this way I was directed back to Sam, and with my hands feeling charged with energy, they were guided to either side of his head, stopping within inches of making contact.***

***"It feels like I can feel all of the static electricity at my head coming from your hands," Sam said.***

***Indeed, I felt it, too. It was like energy was being directed from me to him.***

***"I'm feeling all of these pulsations," he continued. "And it feels like it's doing something."***

***Yes, this was Qi emission – what I'd been leery of and refused to perform for the last thirty years.***

*"I'm feeling the effects are all over my body," he continued. "All the way down to my legs."*

*Over time, the feeling of energy in my hands dissipated, signaling the end of the session.*

*"I really felt something happen with this," Sam declared. "The other time the feeling was subtle, but this time it was really definite. I really felt places in my body where they were healing as a result of this - Where I had healing - And the headache is gone."*

*I stood back stunned: It seemed that when I did that Qi Gong self-practice with the intent of being more helpful to Sam, the Universal Qi recognized that what my friend needed as Qi emission, and being that I was didn't understand how to perform Qi emission, it would essentially 'take me by the hand' and guide me through that process itself...*

That experience forever changed me and my trajectory in Qi Gong. I'd crossed a threshold that enabled me. I could perform chi emission now without a shred of difficulty.

"I can see that your energies resonate," she said. "It seems like you learned more of your energy stuff by interacting with him. I know it's the same thing for other people: If you get two people with similar something... Like, by themselves, they really aren't much. They're not dangerous. Just angry. But when you put them with another type of person who complements them in a different way, then all of a sudden, the two of them are dangerous to society; whereas one alone is not."

Yes, left to my own devices, and I was floundering with Qi Gong; put us together, and Sam gave me the wherewithal to perform Qi Gong at its highest level.

"And I think about that with what you say about Sam and where you learn your energy stuff from," she continued. "Because I'm sure these people around you have taught you - because somehow, they're able to send some of this to you. Maybe even some folks who aren't trained? Like me?"

Yes, she had been the first person who taught me.

*On a summer day my beloved college friend Bubbles and I rode out to the fields beyond the campus, and sitting under the shade of a tree sharing a picnic lunch, exchanged stories from our lives. She described the sad occurrence of a neighborhood girl struck by a drunk driver; the girl had been riding her bike at the time, and when she died, Bubbles' father reacted harshly.*

***"He took our bikes away," Bubbles said. "We were never allowed to ride them again."***

***She broke off and looked away. Gazing at her I knew her father had only acted to try to protect the daughters he loved! But, at the same time, I realized it made her sad.***

***Then, it happened: I forgot myself and all that mattered was my cherished friend; and in that moment, I had a feeling like I'd left my physical body and were existing only in spirit.***

***"I feel for you," I said, reaching out to her. "I feel for you..."***

**"And I don't know what I'm doing and not doing," she continued. "But it just seems like maybe that's what Sam was for you? He's got something that he gives off that helps you to learn and harness what you're doing? Who knows?..."**

# CHAPTER SIXTY

While visiting with Sam, our mutual friend, Dino, came to Sam's home. Dino inquired about Sam's condition? Sam responded with details about his activity tolerance, like that 150 steps was his limit at one time before his oxygen levels dropped.

"It will actually go down after 100 steps," he added. "But you're catching me at a pretty good time."

Sam introduced Dino to his wife. His wife remembered Dino from my birthday, in which we did karaoke.

Sam described how he'd made plans with the lung transplant service to undergo evaluations the week of June 16th.

"So, I'll be going there every day for a week, doing a battery of tests," he said. "And on the last day, I'll be under [general anesthesia], because they said that they were going to perform a cardio test, where they apparently put something in my heart, so I can only assume that it's going to be a little bit more invasive, and more than a finger prick test. Everything seems to be speeding ahead."

Sam said he was trying to avoid stress.

"Because, for me, every breath is a struggle," he said. "I'm already in my sympathetic, fight or flight mode, so anything that adds any more on top of that stress-wise is significant. So, if I can clear my head and take care of even little things that bother me, it's a big deal."

"Mike mentioned that," Dino interjected. "So, I brought over some CBD gummies."

He described how we used them to help him sleep, as well as the different varieties he'd tried.

Sam talked about his experience, saying that in his youth, he tried it and he gave him at best 'the giggles', as opposed to the high that his friends got.

"But I do know that it has a calming effect," Sam said. "So, I thought maybe as things get worse for me and my condition declines here."

"I would suggest that you experiment with them sooner than later," Dino said. "Because maybe this isn't the right combination and there's another one that you'd like to try. Start slow and that way you'll know."

Sam asked if he could pay Dino? Dino was quick to say no.

"This is so nice of you, Dino," Sam said. "I really, really appreciate it. It's really kind of you to consider this."

Sam talked about the drastic changes that he had undergone with his lungs.

"It feels like I dropped off a cliff and I'm down to a ledge, and then I dropped off to another ledge," he said. "And I know that there are more drops to come. So, I'm trying to anticipate, instead of reacting to my drops. Otherwise, that causes even more anxiety when all of a sudden, I'm going, 'Whoa, I'm in unknown territory', versus being more of a Boy Scout, prepared for my next hike."

"It just started in January that I started really declining," Sam said. "Before that, I was able to walk a mile or two miles."

Dino asked if anything precipitated that?

"No, just my lung was getting more fibrotic," he responded.

Oddly, he didn't talk about his bout with the acute COVID-19 infection and then the problems of long Covid?

"Did you get sick or anything?" Dino asked.

"This is what happened," he said. "My sickness is one of my systems slowing down. For instance, when it comes to my appetite, I still want to eat something, but when I start eating it, I feel full. And my stomach feels like it's not doing anything, and the food just sits there.

"And the reason is, I'm in a sympathetic mode. Again, fight or flight. And when you're in that mode, when you're fighting, you're not hungry. In fact, your body tries to say, 'You need to get out of this danger. We're going to try to turn everything towards your muscles.' So, your enzymes in your stomach started to degrade and those amino acids go to your muscles, rather than towards eating.

"And when you're in this sympathetic mode, your stomach doesn't want you to have a lot of peristaltic motion. So, they have slowed down. So, even though I'm saying, 'I need to eat', my system isn't responding. So, I've been losing weight.

"But your weight is OK?" Dino asked.

"No," he responded. "I'm trying to eat a little bit a lot. That's how I'm trying to compensate. And May has been wonderful. She got me these protein drinks, so I've been drinking these protein drinks."

"In one way, this is terrible," Sam concluded. "But in another way, I'm experiencing things that I've never experienced before. So that I'm learning about myself and things that I took for granted..."

Dino said he hoped that the CBD would help with his appetite, as well as calm his nerves.

"You've given me something to experiment with, and I'm really grateful," Sam responded.

Dino asked if Sam was able to enjoy anything at this time?

"Because of this, I've taken up Qi Gong and Tai Chi," Sam responded. "And I'm finding that I'm really enjoying it. I think before, it was harder for me to do these things, because I was so active. So, I was really on adrenaline, and this is so slow and calm. But now I'm in that position where slow and calm is like superfast for me! So, it's perfect and now I can understand it better. And my wife does Qi Gong, so I'm able to do these things with her.

"And I also do Tai Chi, but I don't go to class anymore, because I cough too much, and I think that freaks out everybody, especially in the post-Covid era now. And so, I've been learning it on my own, which I find very enlightening. I learned it more by myself, and even though I make a lot of mistakes, I also find a lot of solutions."

Dino asked if Sam had done anything like this in the past?

"Not Tai Chi or Qi Gong," he said. "I did more of a harder martial arts, like karate, judo and kendo. So, I've had experiences that helped me advance pretty quickly.

"But I'll tell you, there are some things that you can't replace without years of dedicated experience. Because you have to develop those neural systems and pathways, as well as the alignment of the body. And you also have to get the feel of the Chi."

Sam talked about working with the Post Study Long COVID-Qi Gong group.

"Tonight, I'm planning to do that over the phone and follow along with the group," Sam said. "I did that last week, and I found it, even over the phone, that it was stronger when I was working through Mike on this. I've been doing this before, but it felt stronger through Mike. Maybe it's because Mike explains it better?"

Sam indicated that he was going to rest before he did the group of practice with me.

"I get tired quickly," he said, wearily.

**Dino told Sam to call him in a week and give him some feedback.**

**"Hit me up next week," Dino said…**

**Later, Sam was worried about cannabis use, saying that one of the questions in the questionnaire from Stanford's lung transplant service was whether he was on marijuana?**

**"And I'm wondering if marijuana use might exclude me from getting on the lung transplant list?" he queried.**

**"It definitely helped me in the time that I used it," he said. "An hour after I got back from the hospital from coughing up that blood I was feeling edgy, and I took the gummy, and it took away the edge in about half an hour. Maybe less than that. And I thought, 'That was great.'**

**"But the marijuana was like a memory eraser. It just wiped out my memory of how I should be reacting to this incident. I was trying to recall how I felt, and I couldn't recall it? It was like any issue with that feeling was just wiped out - Wiped out of my memory. That's how strong it was. It was just really weird.**

**"And the next day I was thinking, 'You know, I wonder if this would help me with my appetite?' So that morning, I decided to take the other half, and I ate breakfast, and I noticed that I was eating a little bit more. So, it might've helped me with my appetite, too.**

**"And then I just stopped because of the questions about marijuana. I'll ask them about that this week, because I have to call them up. So, for the meantime, I haven't taken anymore..."**

# CHAPTER SIXTY-ONE

Wednesday, May 28, 2025
Long COVID-Qi Gong post study group.

Prior to Sam calling in to participate in the self-practice portion of the Qi Gong practice, I performed external Qi Gong with the members of the group.

I worked with Ruth first: It felt like there was this energy spray that was coming off of her and bouncing off of my hand into the heavens.

Ruth described, feeling like there was this large amount of energy coming out from her, like a volcano, and she was enjoying being immersed in what felt like a sea of energy.

Indeed, Rosa described being able to see that energy, leaving ruth as though it were like vapor coming from her.

"Like you were the wicked witch from the Wizard of Oz," she said.

Ruth laughed.

With Rosa, it was a more standard interaction of feeling the energy around her chest area, until I felt this energy at my third eye that extended to my upper scalp and down to the tip of my nose.

When I described my energy experience, she indicated that that was in the same area that she was experiencing that pressure on her face that felt like I had my hand there. I wondered if there were some activation of pressure receptors with the energy experience, just as Sam described when he was talking about energy acting at some physical level?

I was standing with my head directed downwards and wondered if my energy was perhaps in line and interacting with Rosa's, but I didn't know where I was because my eyes were closed. I asked Ruth if it looked like my third eye was directed in the same plane as Rosa's third eye? Ruth affirmed that it was…

When we were ready for the self-practice, I called Sam to join us. During the self-practice, Sam said his hands moved apart from 6 inches to about a foot and stayed there. He described how his hands were at the level of his chest, and there was an energy at his head, he said, and he thought that was because it made sense that his hands were charged and full of energy and near his chest, because that's where he needed it for his lungs.

Ruth remarked that Sam had stopped coughing during the self-practice, and Sam described his ease of breathing.

I hoped that this practice was giving him the parasympathetic stimulation and consequent ease that he was looking for.

Then, Sam offered his thoughts about the self-practice.

"I think that anything that moves you more to parasympathetic mode gets you towards more fertile ground to enjoy Qi Gong and your energy," he began. "So, anything in your environment that helps that is beneficial. And I think you can feel the emotions of the people who surround you, so that if everyone around you is calm and collected and engaged in a more parasympathetic mode themselves, then your environment around you is a lot more relaxing and calming and engaging the parasympathetic responses in your feelings.

"I think the intensity of you're doing energy and Qi Gong, which most people call it the energy of chi, but I think a lot of it is biologic responses, too. Just like when someone talks to you in a soft, calm voice, you're more relaxed, and your body is less tense. And I think your blood flow increases because you're not constricting vessels in your body because of the sympathetic nervous system. All that aid in the flow of blood, and as part of the chi, so that you're much more likely to feel the energy of chi.

"So, I think that doing this with all three of you really helps out, providing a very nice environment for me to experience myself fuller…"

"I also think we're focusing on the now," Rosa added. "I'm not thinking about paying my bills the way I was earlier. I'm focusing on what I'm doing right now and how I'm breathing and sensing my body."

"Yes, I think that's very important," Sam said. "I always said that the beauty of skiing is that when you're on the slopes, you don't think about the problems you have in the valley. You're only thinking about the present and the enjoyment you're having by skiing down the mountain."

It happened that I was in a deep Qi Gong state with my axial skeleton moving about my pelvic bowl again.

"Dancing in your chair," ruth commented.

"Like a mortar and pestle," Sam added.

Yes, and it seemed to have a very good effect on me by stretching the tight muscles in my sacroiliac region.

I told Sam about my feelings of being in sympathetic overload during my time of being homeless after the Yale plans broke down and that constant cold sweat I experienced down my spine.

"Well, it's important to re-center yourself," he responded. "And when you're able to find that center again, you're able to be in a calmer, in parasympathetic mode, and able to think clearly and basically feel like you're starting anew. And that now is the beginning to really take on things again."

"Grow anew," I thought. It was something from a dream I'd after leaving LA County USC Neurology and finally getting myself out of a persistent state of stress and disappointment...

I asked how Sam was doing? And whether he was in that place of 'starting anew' and feeling ready to take on the challenges of the lung transplant evaluations?

"I'm just trying to optimize my situation where it is currently," he responded. "The operation will come when it comes, and then I'll deal with it at the time.

"Of course, you want to be a good Boy Scout and prepare for every eventuality. But that's the best you can do - is just prepare.

"But you're not at the campsite yet. And there's going to be a lot of unexpected things in between.

"But if you're prepared enough, you'll be able to take it on.

"But you shouldn't have to sweat the details. You should just try to be prepared and work on your current situation where you're at. Because if you don't, you're going to have to move on without something that's been resolved. And then you carry that unresolved issue forward, and that's only going to drag you down. So, it's best that your preparation deals with optimizing the current situation.

"So, that's what I'm doing. I'm making myself as healthy as I can. That's like preparing and also enjoying the optimization of today and also preparing myself so that I can survive the surgery in the best way.

"So, it's really important to do both - Optimize and prepare.

**"But optimization is the most important thing, because when you're optimized, you can do more. And if you do more, then you can prepare more. You can take on challenges in the best way that you possibly can. And you might not be able to do things that you used to do in your current situation, so you have to figure out how best you can do things in your current condition. And how you can, again, calm down and be as prepared and make yourself as strong as you possibly can under the conditions that you're under."**

**"That's pretty much what I'm focused on," he concluded…**

**I asked Sam if we should let him get some rest? He agreed and got off the call.**

**Ruth commented about the healing effect that Sam seemed to have on me.**

**"Sam does seem to have energized you these last couple of times, Dr. Mike," she commented.**

**Yes, I felt for Sam a keen feeling of kinship, like we were a couple of blind men, trying to navigate this unknown and uncharted energetic space, and happy because we like to explore...**

# CHAPTER SIXTY-TWO

Where Sam had raised the question about whether performing the self-practice in a larger group is more beneficial, I reached out to ChiSing, who was a member of my original Qi Gong group (from thirty years ago in DC) for a potential answer.

"According to Master Chou, each person alone puts out so much energy into the compassion field," she said. "So, if two people practice, it becomes twice as strong. Three, three-fold. 10, 10-fold the energy - That's ten times as much as if you practice alone."

I shared how it was that Sam had effectively intuited this since joining our Qi Gong self-practices and had commented that the energy felt stronger and wondered if it was because it involved more people?

"Yeah, absolutely," she responded. "You get an amplification…"

I called Sam and shared ChiSing's comments. He agreed.

"When I feel that Qi in the group, the Qi is stronger," he said. "And as things were moving from my chest, down my arms, to my hands, it seemed like it left my fingers and went to the ground."

Sam added that he felt he was doing better.

"And I attribute that to the session of chi gong that I did with you," he said. "There just seems like there's the connection there."

"Please take it with a grain of salt," he added, "but if I was going to say that there was one thing that helped me the most, it was your Qi Gong session over the phone. After that, I felt like I was able to do more exercise, which I thought was improving my endurance, stamina and strength. I'm noticing that my recovery time for my O2 level and heart rate is better. So, thank you for that session. I just felt so relaxed. If anything, it got me to a good place..."

Before Sam got off the phone, he told me about plans for the lung transplant.

"I didn't know that you could be spending three months at Stanford Hospital after the surgery," he began, "and in the beginning, I'll be on dialysis and heart monitor, because my system would be debilitated and need recover. They showed me a picture of a person with equipment all around him.

"And then they said you have to take 40 pills a day for the rest of your life. And you have to take them precisely accurately, because you can't have ups and downs on your levels.

"So, it's really regimented. It would be easier if I climbed Mount Everest without oxygen than to live like this. But in the time that you do have, if you get this procedure, you can move around and do things. So, I guess that's worth it.

"And they went over the statistics. It's a little bit worse than what you read. Rather than 90% that survive the first year, it was closer to 80%. And instead of a five-year survival rate, they gave a three year and that dropped."

Then, he indicated that he had to take an incoming call.

"I'm sorry that my time is being so taken by nurses and visitors," he said. "Just every day. Everybody's trying to get me ready, which is nice…"

Getting off the phone with Sam, I had a moment of weakness, in which I considered my own age and condition and wondered if it wasn't too late for me to be doing this research fellowship and effectively looking to change careers at this stage of my life?

"You're not 18," April said. "If you were 18, it would be different."

Yes. Indeed, I was already some five years older than when my father retired.

I do have a feeling like this project can be successful. And every time I perform BioEnerQi, it feels like a miracle… Just feeling this invisible source of energy from somebody's energetic circulation and finding an energy disturbance and connecting with it and moving with it and being directed by it… It all feels like a miracle.

However, given that I have no way of explaining or quantitating or measuring what's going on, isn't it an unfair burden on that other person?...

During the night, I dreamt a young, more compact and smaller Abraham Lincoln came to lead the people.

And whereas I went to bed feeling tight in my chest, I awoke with a feeling like it was wide open.

Abraham Lincoln had been my role model in childhood. I am compact and smaller than Lincoln. My chest is where I hold my stress, and waking up as I had showed me that it's within my power for my chest to be open, and it being closed down is likely mostly the result of something I'm doing mentally.

"And you don't want to be stuck," my therapist asserted. "You don't want to be stagnant. You want to follow your heart and do your life's work..."

"What a dream!" my therapist commented. "To build the field that you're involved in. And merge east and west. So many people like to polarize things. But I don't think they have to be. I feel like your work is a blending of eastern and western. Because you have the background in both. You've seen both of them work. You're willing to work with both of them.

"And you've back it up with something. With the clinical study that you carried out. If you could have more research, you could carry on this work and train others to do so..."

Meanwhile, I was becoming more concerned about Sam: The other day, he'd called sounding more breathless than I'd ever heard him. He said he was doing a lot of work to clear his storage spaces. Indeed, a cousin who had been working with him had a heart attack while helping him, and this was weighing heavily on Sam.

In addition to all that, a colonoscopy had been scheduled for him, as among the hurdles that he had to clear for the lung transplant evaluations.

"They rushed this," he said. "They had a cancellation, and I had to call the doctors, and I just barely got the solution that you have to drink an hour ago. So, I have to take it when they offer it to me and that's sooner than later."

Just then, a call came in from the hospital, probably about his cousin with the heart attack, and Sam insisted he had to get off and take it...

# CHAPTER SIXTY-THREE

Wednesday, June 4, 2025
Long COVID-Qi Gong post study group.

Working with Rosa, it felt like energy coming from the upper chakras, like a strong breeze blowing against my hand, they kept on getting bigger and wider, so that I could feel it between my hands, starting with a smaller diameter of about 6 to 8 inches, And then expanding like a trunk of a giant tree that kept on expanding.

I felt my crown chakra open, and the energy connecting at my solar plexus, as well as there being this feeling of energy coming from my dantian.

"I experienced a lot of warmth in my hands," Rosa said. "And I felt energy radiating through my body up to my throat area. And then I felt a sharp discomfort, like a blade. But not really painful. Just a blade feeling. And then it went up and out through my hands. And the discomfort went away."

I thought about Sam's knife analogy...

In the Qi Gong self-practice that followed, Sam reported that feelings in his lungs of energy had moved outwards down his arms into his hands, and then into the ground.

"I felt like energy was radiating from that area through my hands," he said. "It's really interesting… Earlier this week I felt chest pain. And they were just light, and I don't know if there's any relationship between what I was feeling in my throat? I'm actually feeling really good now."

I thought that sounded healing.

"It is," he responded. "Because my chest feels very relaxed."

I asked how he had been doing for these past days?

"Overall, I feel a little bit better compared to last week," he replied. "I think the things that I've been doing have been optimizing my breathing for my condition. I think one of the nice things about this is that it makes us more sensitive and more aware of our bodies."

Then, he cautioned Rosa to get herself checked out for chest pain.

"Because it might be a very early warning sign of something that might be coming," he said. "I just wouldn't want anything to happen to you."

I explained that it was Sam and my strong opinion that folk should have everything checked out before they initiated by energy treatments, because these treatments inherently make people feel good in general, maybe because they do activate the parasympathetic, etc., and that could be risky if they have some underlying medical condition, and that it might give them a false sense of security and therefore potentially lead to a delay in care.

Then, I asked Rosa if she had been thoroughly checked out before the Qi Gong study, as I imagine that she had been?

Rosa responded that her heart was being monitored carefully.

"By a long Covid doctor and by regular physicians," she said. "The heart issue is ongoing. I have palpitations on a regular basis. I've been instructed that if my heart rate exceeds 200 bpm, I'm to immediately go to the ER. I've only had to do that a couple of times."

"So, I've been thoroughly monitored," she concluded. "It's just the long Covid messing with my body..."

Sam described his ongoing issues and symptoms of long Covid.

"I think my symptoms of long Covid are diminishing," he said, "but of course my lung issues are getting worse.

"When I had my long Covid symptoms, there was a huge change in being lethargic - Lots of malaise and such, so that I just couldn't move at all. And that was different than just because of my lungs.

"Of course, I had difficulty breathing at the time, and that didn't help my energy, as well. But my energy with long Covid was such that my muscles just weren't working.

"And now my muscles are working. But there's no endurance in me. And between that and losing weight and losing muscle mass, that's making me weak now. It isn't long Covid anymore, as much as from the effects of the interstitial lung disease and all of its ramifications in weight loss and muscle loss and no energy because of not having oxygen.

"It was like I replaced one damaging thing with another damaging thing," he concluded…

Rosa talked about her recent bout with a respiratory infection, that went onto shingles, as well as issues with her ears and vertigo.

"And I never had all of these things happen to me," she said. "And it took me months to heal.

"And when I was talking with my doctor about this, it was his thought that the long Covid may have done something to my immune system, where I'm more susceptible and have difficulties healing."

"Yes, isn't it amazing this long Covid and all of its cascading effects and what it can do to our bodies?" Sam began. "It's really hard to explain all of this to someone who's never experienced this. It's like driving a car, and all of a sudden, it's not just one issue that goes wrong with the car, it's all kinds: the engine's not running; you have a cracked frame; you can't roll the windows down; the heater and air conditioning aren't working; the wheels are falling off; you can't even adjust your seat.

"And you can deal with it when there's just one problem - You can get that fixed - Bring it into the service department and have them fix it.

"But not when everything is falling apart. Then people just look at it and say, 'Oh, no, that goes into the scrap heap'…

"But people don't realize that," Sam continued, after having essentially perfectly captured how these patients were feeling as they struggled in the medical system. "I've heard lots of people with long Covid try to explain it to family members, and the family members just can't believe it. They think you're just lazy."

Rosa agreed.

"Exactly," she said. "Until I came into the support group here, I really felt alienated from my family. I got tired of telling them how I was feeling, because they would look at me and say, 'Maybe you're just getting old?'"

"That's a real good catch-all phrase," Sam responded. "'Yeah, you're getting old'."

Rosa described how active she'd been before acquiring long Covid.

"I was doing weightlifting," she said. "And then everything stopped. In fact, just this week, I was sitting in my chair and felt good enough to go back to lifting weights. And I haven't felt good enough to do that in a long, long time."

"It's devastating," she concluded. "You don't even know yourself. You go, 'Who am I now?'…

Sam intuited that Rosa had been athletic.

"It sounds like before long Covid, you had been very strong," he said.

"Oh, yeah," Rosa responded. "I used to ride bikes. I used to do the Centennial's. I was very fit. Right before Covid, I had my own personal trainer. And then Covid happened, and all this got shut down. I was thinking about how I would ride my bike in the Centennial, and I would get to the last few miles, and I would get that runners high, and you couldn't stop me. I was just going. Going right past the finish line.

"So, I was thinking there must be some correlation between runners high and that energy release? Because that's what it felt like. Like a big release. And you couldn't stop me. I was like a rocket. Like a rocket taking off for the finish line."

"I can tell that you're a very good athlete," Sam said. "And I hope you'll get back to a state that will help you get great joy."

"And I had a lot of depression that I had to work through over the past years," Rosa confided. "Just because I can't do those things.

"But I've come to appreciate where I'm at now and honor what I can do."

"I think Tai Chi will be very good for you," Sam said. "I think you'll feel it sooner than most people. And I think your agility that you had once will come back very quickly, and you'll be able to perform the Tai Chi better than your average person. I think you'll feel really good when you get into it. You might feel discouraged in the beginning, because you're going to find that it's a lot more complicated than people just making all of these movements that look so graceful and easy. Because it's not."

"So, it takes a while," he concluded, "but you're an athlete and you know how to work it…"

# CHAPTER SIXTY-FOUR

Sunday, June 8, 2025

Sam called and told me that the night before, he'd required emergency attention for choking and coughing blood.

"I couldn't breathe," he explained. "It happened when I had a sip of water, and it got caught in my throat… I wanted to expel it out, and of course, my lungs don't have that much expiration capability.

"I was finally able to cough, and when I did cough, blood came out. Had blood not come out, I wouldn't have gone to the emergency room.

"I guess I'm getting used to it, because I didn't panic as much as I did the first time. But I still panicked. So, I told my wife, 'Because of the bleeding, I think we should go to the emergency room, just in case. Because if it's going to continue to bleed, I don't want to be laying there asleep and drown in my own blood.'

"The blood was bright red, so it wasn't from the lung.

"In the emergency room, they did all these tests… CT and x-rays and blood test, and they basically came to the conclusion that my condition hasn't changed significantly, and the bleeding was from my throat.

"And they didn't think of something that was really serious. They just said, 'You probably have been irritating that quite a bit, and it finally got irritated enough to bleed'…"

I hurried to Sam's. When I arrived, he repeated about treating the planned lung transplant as his expedition up Mount Everest.

"Instead of looking at it like, 'This is terrible. I'm going to be in a lot of pain. It's going to be frightening, and the risk and the side effects can be terrible', I'm going, 'Look, if I was an astronaut and I was going to go up into space, you've got to be able to make it. And it requires technology.'

"So, I decided, 'Look, you're fortunate', and instead of looking at each catheterization as a painful, inconvenient thing, I have to look at it like, 'This is what it takes to climb that summit. And this is my new adventure in life. And I've got to see how I can withstand this adventure.'

"And maybe the side effects won't be terrible, and I won't have those bad side effects. And just like in any expedition, if you get these bad side effects, you weren't meant to make it to the top. But let's see how close I can get to the top. This will be a nice challenge.

"I mean, since I have to do it anyways, I might as well make it a challenge and see if I can get through it? Because if I do get through it, I'll be in a healthier state."

He described how it was that just before I arrived, he had his family over and had difficulty escorting them outside to say goodbye.

"I thought, 'This is difficult. I just need to get back in the house and sit. Well, if the lung transplant worked, I'd be able to walk out several times before I felt that way. Maybe even walk and hike.'

"And then, I thought, 'I'd have to take a lot of medications, maybe I'd have to do this and that?' But that's part of the challenge. I'm going to be on the expedition for the rest of my life. I have to keep climbing Mount Everest several times in my lifetime.

"But it would be exciting to summit!

"Right now, I'm getting to base one. Base Two. And base seven is very critical."

"Anyway," he concluded, "we'll see…"

Before starting the external Qi Gong, I suggested we have a conversation about what we were looking to achieve? What his intention would be? What would be our focus if we could choose to focus on something? If it was something that we could direct our efforts and energies towards - and the sky was the limit - what would it be? How would Qi Gong help him best? If we could say there was no limit to the benefit that Qi Gong could give him? If anything was possible? If all possibilities were on the table? And could we approach it that way? If we could "go for broke"? Go for curing this thing and addressing it at its root cause?

If so, what would be our goal in this session and the sessions to come? What would be the optimal? The ultimate in healing that we could imagine be achieved? And how could we let that direct how we would go into this Qi Gong session? What if we approached it that way and tried? We asked for it all, in other words? What would that look like?

I said that when it came to his difficulties of long Covid, my intention had been to recharge his batteries.

"And that happened to an extent," Sam responded. "I don't think it completely disappeared, but it was less. If I were back in September, I'd still want to be in bed. But now I'm moving about, and I'm feeling like my lungs are the primary thing that's stopping me or slowing me down.

"Before it was my legs and my arms and just all over my body, it was just feeling limp. Like I had no strength at all. My mind was in a fog. That was the Covid. I truly believe that. That was the Covid, because as soon as I got that second Covid... Well, Mike, before that, I was doing all these physical things. I was ramping up on my physical abilities. I was using weights. I was using the bands. I was thinking, 'Man, I'm going to recover from this.'

"But after the Covid, I had no strength... In my arms or legs. But it was a different weakness. It wasn't coming from my lungs then. But the Covid had weakened me. So, it was a difficult transition.

"So, I wasn't even thinking about my lungs... Until I went to see the pulmonologist. I mean, I knew I had interstitial lung disease, but I really didn't understand it. To be honest with you, I was very naïve prior to that. When they initially told me the results of that CT, I thought, 'Oh, I have interstitial lung disease. That doesn't sound so bad.' But then in May, all of a sudden, I couldn't do the six-minute walk. And like I said, it felt like falling off a cliff. Now it's all about my lungs.

"So, talking about the Covid, I just had to find a way to overcome that, and you helped me a lot. I think the sessions we had were helping me get to that point. However, now, it's overlapping with the rising interstitial lung disease. So, it's sort of like an absorption spectrum: If something also absorbs at that wavelength, it covers up your target of absorption.

"I worked on the quantitative absorption of marijuana, and at different levels of the analysis that we were looking for it, it would attach onto this marker, and the marker would be regained as you separated the solution. And so, the more concentrated your target was, the more absorption you saw.

"So, with marijuana alone, we could tell the level of marijuana with the level of THC; however, if you took salicylic acid (aspirin), it also absorbed at the same wavelength. And it would mask the THC. So, if you took salicylic acid, the absorption at that wavelength was so high that you couldn't see the rate change - And we were measuring rate changes. So, therefore, it gave a false negative, because you wouldn't be able to see the rate change. It was covered up by the aspirin.

"So, to get out of a positive marijuana test, you could take aspirin. Because even though you were high on marijuana, if you just took an aspirin, you wouldn't be able to see the rate change of the THC.

"So, what I'm trying to say is, Covid was like the aspirin, and my lungs were trying to show the rate change, but you couldn't see what was happening with my lungs at the beginning because the Covid was overwhelming it."

"But now the long Covid has gone down," he concluded, "and what's replaced it is my lung situation."

Perhaps? I responded. But perhaps it was a continuum, and the Covid had acted to accelerate the autoimmune process that was the basis of the interstitial lung disease?

Nevertheless, the question remained: What could we do? If this were a perfect world, and Qi Gong was a perfect remedy, how could it help him best? In other words, how did the lung condition get worse? Could it be treated at the root cause?

"I like that," Sam said. "You're right. OK, if you look at this post oximeter, I don't need supplemental oxygen for minimal activity. However, the interstitial lung disease is causing stress on me. I think that's because I'm moving into sympathetic activity from parasympathetic activity, and so my system is probably releasing a lot of adrenaline. And with all of this increased activity of a sympathetic, that's probably why this Qi Gong and Tai Chi is very helpful. Because it tries to move me into a more parasympathetic state."

"So, I'm thinking that what you're doing is very much parasympathetic oriented," he concluded. "And I think that's what's been helping me..."

Perhaps I should have been satisfied with Sam was looking for simply inhibition of sympathetic activity and increased parasympathetic activity; however, I persisted and commented that it seemed to me that the physiology we were attempting to combat was autoimmune scarring of the lungs, and if the body could produce such scarring, why can't it reverse it?

"Sure, the fibrolytic system," Sam responded, without hesitation. "Fibrolysis."

He wondered if his aging might be part of it?

"So, I wonder if I could make it back to a more elastic stage and state?" he asked.

He also wondered about the state of his autonomic nervous system in all this?

"I definitely think that when you're in parasympathetic mode, you're not going to be building things up," he said. "I think the parasympathetic state allows more for healing than the sympathetic.

"The sympathetic is putting more stress on the body, so that it's more active and it's short-term; whereas, once you get to a parasympathetic state, you can sleep better, you can do the healing process is more, it allows time for construction to occur, or repair.

"And that's what you do! I mean, when you're doing this, the first thing I always notice... And also the last thing I notice in our sessions... Is that I get very relaxed. I feel good. I feel more sensitive to my surroundings. And there's an awareness to tingling and things like that, where my muscles are expanding or contracting... I can feel all those things. I'm a lot more sensitive.

"And that's very much like internal qi Gong, where you can start feeling all that.

"But it starts with your external Qi gong... Because you can feel the Chi, and your body opens up. You can feel the flow in your capillaries. You can feel your blood flow. You could probably feel your lymphatic system flowing. And I think all that helps aid healing."

Yes, he was exactly right. But I still wanted to drive home the point; that is, what was the ultimate that we could achieve in the session that would help him? For me it was achieving fibrinolysis for him, particularly in his lungs.

I said that for me, my internal Qi Gong practice had moved to the muscular releases and flopping. So that it was bang, bang, bang, bang-bang when it came to these massive muscular releases, opening me up at my chest and solar plexus. What's involved in that? I think it's some kind of charge to get the actin and myosin fibers to unhinged.

"You release the ratchet," Sam commented. "Because it's ratcheting ... Click, click, click, click... and contracting till you release it."

Yes, exactly. That's exactly what's occurring. as usual Sam was exactly right.

I went on and offered the example of kino: With him, it helped him overcome neurologic deficits. How did it do that? What did it do there? I held that it woke up nerves that had been stunned by his traumatic brain injury, and put themselves into a suspended state of animation, so that they were no longer functioning so they could keep themselves at rest and better survive.

Just like what happened to me when I nearly drowned. I was put into the suspended state of animation so that I wouldn't consume as much energy while I was waiting for that lifeguard to pull me out. It gave me a chance to survive.

But now, the blood and nutrients were getting to those nerves. They no longer needed to be in that suspended state of animation. So, what I had to do was give them the wake-up call when it came to that and get them back to functioning.

"Maybe increase the blood flow to certain areas?" Sam suggested. "And really enhance the nerve activity at that site. Because nerve function really relies on a lot of nutrients and oxygen and gas exchange. And, so, by opening it up in particular areas, where maybe it was starving a bit, that's how Kino got better?"

Perhaps, though I still held that it was some rebooting process that got those nerves working again and thought that it was a process not unlike what happens with stroke involving the ischemic penumbra, where the tissue is in that border region of merely dying because of the lack of blood flow, but was able to survive, and just needs some encouragement, essentially to go back to life.

"Basically, it went into life support mode," Sam again expertly diagnosed. "In life support mode, you just have to lay there and survive. But afterwards, we need to be active. So, when you release it, everything just starts flowing, and it goes, 'Oh, I'm alive again.' Meaning, 'I can move.' Before that, it's approach had been, 'I have to conserve myself. I have to be still and do the minimal in activity as possible. I am on life support.' Just like a submarine crew when they're running out of oxygen. Or in a space capsule, and they moved to life-support."

Yes, but for some reason, the body didn't recognize that Kino was ready to come out of that life support mode and suspended an animation; it needed the external Qi Gong to flip that switch and wake it up.

"I think it's very complex," Sam said. "It's not just one thing that has to work right. It's probably a whole handful of things, or series of things that has to happen. It's sort of like switching on a sequence: You can't just turn all the switches on; you have to throw this switch, and then that switch.

"And so maybe that's what Qi Gong does. It knows the code, or the sequence, that is required to awaken the system?"

Yes, like the code for awakening the frozen release system.

Or maybe it was really simple, and the Qi Gong just flipped one switch and that triggers the flipping of all the others. Who knows?

"Yes," Sam said. "It could have been that most all of the switches were on, and there were just a few that weren't, and your Qi Gong hit the right ones. Who knows?

"But when we come back to here, what's the best way to get my session so that it maximizes all of this waking up, so to speak?..."

"I can tell you that my most limited system is, I feel out of breath," Sam said. "I feel pressure from the chest that just sort of radiates to the rest of the body and makes me feel very tired. So, I guess anything that would help minimize that.

"And I think that involves two things: one is a mental component, because I know that when I'm distracted, I feel pretty good; and if my mind starts to focus too much on my problems, I think I make it worse. And distraction is probably how THC works, too. It distracts and doesn't allow me to think about that issue.

"And then there's the second one, which is the physical aspects of the strain of my lungs trying to expand: I try to blow into that peak flow meter, and the best I can do is 250 now. And I dropped down to 200 sometimes. So that's my next limiting thing: my battle with a negative pressure in my thoracic cavity. I can raise and lower my diaphragm, but the lung just doesn't inflate. So, it's fighting that. so that's the second thing that's draining me that I can imagine.

"So, thinking about it, my subconscious doesn't help me, and the strain of the muscles in my chest, and the diaphragm is probably the next thing. And that affects all the rest of my movements."

But this didn't have anything to do specifically with fibrinolysis. As such, I tried to bring Sam back to that, imagining it was the ultimate that we might be able to achieve - The Hail Mary - and focus on whatever it was that caused his system to produce scarring and send a message that it no longer needed to do it.

"You got the asbestos out of the house," I said. "You're not exposing yourself to the silicon on the ski deck"

"Or the rug fibers," Sam added. "And I tried to minimize going outside to expose myself to allergens."

"And you don't have an active TB infection for the system to react against," I added.

"And I'm not working with chemicals that are toxic," Sam said.

Yes, so all of these things that his body previously might have had a reason to react against and cover up so to produce scarring, we're no longer there. So, there was no reason for the body to do that anymore - There was nothing for it to plaster down and scar over anymore for the purpose of protecting itself. There isn't the silicon, there isn't asbestos, there isn't a TB infection, there isn't the rug fibers, etc.

And there was every reason for the body to let go of the scarring and, instead, promote fibrinolysis - because that's what he needed to live! His system needed to reverse the scarring and restore his health.

"Sure, correct," Sam responded. "So, you're thinking that I could stop the process, there's a good chance of stopping it from getting worse?" he said.

I didn't know that he could 'stop the process.' I was just talking about 'the ultimate' in giving him back his health.

Indeed, the ultimate was more than just stopping the process - The ultimate was reversing it with fibrinolysis.

"But now, how do I reverse it, so I can get a little more capability?" he asked.

It would be fibrinolysis, I responded. The process of reversing the scarring.

"Breaking up the fibrin," he correctly deduced. "Breaking up the scars."

Yes, that would be the penultimate when it came to the body working to self-heal from this condition…

Sam turned to a discussion of the fibrinolysis medication.

"That is very expensive," he said. "The pharmacist I believe was saying it's $2000 a treatment. But if it works, it's better than a lung transplant. My insurance is battling that out right now with the pharmacy."

Then, Sam talked about the nebulizer.

"But even that is working less than less," he said, "and I find that I'm straining just sitting there and breathing it in and out."

That may be, I interrupted. But what I want to focus on here was what Qi Gong might be able to achieve, harnessing Qi Gong to address the root of illness.

If the medication would help the body do this, then great. Right now, though, I want to focus on what Qi Gong might be able to do - If Qi Gong could facilitate the body in some process to help heal itself, I think that fibrinolysis would be the best process for it to help.

"Oh, yeah, that's where I think our focus needs to be, here," Sam affirmed. "I agree. The other stuff… Well, great if it could happen. But the best would be if the body would do it on its own."

"So, what conclusion are you coming up with now?" he asked.

I said that we had a goal. Now the question was how and if we could facilitate it?...

Next, was to answer the question of whether it would be better to do this with him sitting up or laying down?

"Well, I have this massage table," he said. "We could open it up. And if you want me to lay on it, it would be better than on the ground, I guess. Let's try it..."

With Sam on the massage table, I scanned him energetically. To my surprise, I didn't feel much in the way of energy until my hand was really close to his body, like some 6 to 8 inches away. This was surprising, because these days I typically "plug into" folks' energy from well over a foot away?

It felt like maybe there was some sense of energy from further away, but it was really weak, at the threshold of my ability to perceive.

It started with my right hand near his right shoulder, and moved my hand along the surface of his body inches away from his skin, so that I was worried that I was going to make physical contact, especially as these days I prefer to keep my eyes closed during these energy sessions.

And the energy that I was perceiving wasn't usual. It was not a breeze. Instead, it was thousands of infinitesimal electrical impulses against the palm of my hand.

My head became activated with energy, but it was more around my upper third eye/scalp. and that felt different, too. It was like I was wearing a helmet that boxers wear, so that there was the band of energy around my scalp, and another one over the top of my head.

And the energy that I was feeling over my head wasn't all that different from the way I was feeling it at my right hand. It felt like all of these charged impulses at my head.

This was all unusual. And it wasn't the usual pleasant 'awe and reverence' that I typically perceive in these energy exchanges. It wasn't a cocoon of energy. This was all crazy electrical. It felt like I was wearing some 'master of the universe' helmet, conducting some intergalactic war in my mind, like in 'Ender's Gam', a science fiction movie that I once watched in which a young boy saves the universe.

It all seemed to suggest that my mind was working at some level of intricate detail like I'd never worked with anyone before. Like everything before had been simple, child's play compared to this; whereas this seemed to involve thousands of circuits being switched, as opposed to the relaxed 'scan and plug in' that usually happened.

The energy sent me slowly moving around Sam as he lay on the massage table - Millimeter by millimeter.

Then, it finally held me by Sam's left arm/shoulder and wouldn't let me go anywhere, while this net of electrical impulses continued to interact with my hand.

And even though it was my right hand that was the one that was in contact with Sam through all of this, I was feeling a less intense feeling of electrical impulses in my left hand, with the same feeling of electrical circuitry.

And my left hand wanted to be extended at the wrist just like my right hand (palms down)...

At minute five, the intensity of the electrical impulses subsided. There weren't quite the pops everywhere, though at my head, there was still that interesting boxer helmet configuration of electrical charge across my scalp and the top of my head.

My hands were directed off to the right as though I were holding some slender oval shaped energy ball that was full of charge. It was moving down towards the ground, but on the way, it was interacting with my abductor muscles at my groin, so I could feel the charge going to my legs.

I kneeled and followed the energy downwards. I wasn't willing to go down to my knees until it made me do so…

At minute eight, the energy was out of my hands, and all in my head, mostly at my upper third eye. My hands were on the ground.

Sam was giving off these sounds of struggling to breathe, as though grunting. I thought about telling Sam that it would be OK for him to change his position if it would make this easier for him, but decide against it, because the energy experience was so intense that I felt I just had to let Sam do whatever he needed…

At minute nine, Sam's struggling and grunting was getting louder; but the energy was becoming more and more intense at my forehead, so that I couldn't so much as move it: I couldn't lift my head up. It wouldn't let me. It was like I was connected with a "tractor beam" between my head and where I could hear Sam, so that there was this beam of energy that was resisting my moving my head, and I couldn't move my head anywhere now.

The energy of my upper third eye was connected with Sam somehow and either sending energy to him or just held there by this energy tractor beam…

At minute ten, Sam continued to grunt and offer expiratory gasps. And I still couldn't move my head: Every time I try to adjust it and lift it a little, the energy basically said no and resisted. My head was simply being held in place there, and it felt like there was some energy tractor beam between Sam and me.

And I couldn't tell if I was beaming energy at Sam? My head was just being energetically held in place with a feeling of all this electrical impulse energy at the front of my scalp.

It felt like Qi emission coming directly from my head - From my upper third eye…

At minute 11, finally, that feeling of having a tractor beam holding my head let go, so that my head was now just full of energy, though mostly at the upper third eye.

So, Sam, that's it," I said. "If you've been struggling to maintain your supine position on the massage table, you can do whatever is comfortable now. Where are you at?"

No response. And he was silent and not grunting anymore and asleep on the massage table.

At the exact same moment that I'm done, it turns out that he's done! I thought.

He remained asleep for another five minutes and probably only awoke because I was talking into my voice recorder.

"I was relaxed," Sam said. "It felt good."

I shared my thoughts as pertained to the session, especially as it left me to recall an experience from 30 years ago at Dr. Rind's clinic in which I was working with a child with autism and while I was performing bio energy with him, his mother commented that she could see the merging of our auras, so that she felt there was this vast energetic communication happening between us.

"And she saw it with you?" Sam asked.

Yes, in the energetic interaction with her son.

"Could you feel it?" he asked.

No, I couldn't sense anything out of the ordinary then, I said. But what I experienced with Sam just now made me think about that, because it felt like I was connected with his entire nervous system.

"Well, you've been doing it with me for a while," he said. "So, you would notice if it was different."

Yes, it was really different: If ever there were neural activity and a significant exchange happening between myself and someone else (like that woman said she saw between me and her son), this is what it felt like.

I told Sam it just felt like I was connected with his whole nervous system. His energetic system. Like I've never felt an energetic system before.

"All I know is, I was dreaming," he said. "I was dreaming I was at a group luncheon, with all these warming trays with food in them. And I was trying to get food onto my plate. I was totally oblivious of what you were doing. I was just restful sleeping and having a dream."

"The only thing I could feel was around my head," he commented. "How long did we do this for? For about five minutes?"

No, it was 13 minutes of treatment; and then, he was asleep for about just as long before he awoke.

"Yeah, I was totally oblivious to where I was and what you were doing," he said. "I heard you at the beginning. The last thing I remember you say was that it wasn't like you were feeling a strong connection. At the very beginning, it sounded like you had to get really close, and you were right here. And you were moving around. Then, all of a sudden, I didn't hear you. Not at all."

That amounted to about the first 30 seconds of the treatment.

"So, you were talking all that time?" he asked. "Well, I didn't even notice. I only heard you at the very beginning, but I was oblivious after that. I was just into the dream.

"I was trying to scoop up food and put it in my plate. And I couldn't do it. I would scoop out food, and I would pour it into the plate. But only a trickle of food would come out from the spoon - the ladle. It was very disturbing. That I didn't get anything. And I was hungry. And the food was not bad, but I couldn't get it onto the plate."

I told him that I'd been worried, because he was grunting until just as the session ended. Before then, I was feeling this really intense energy connection, and it wasn't until that feeling of being connected by a tractor beam was done that his breathing relaxed and there was no struggling anymore.

"Really?!" he responded. "That is very interesting."

I had made a video at about minute 20 while he was resting comfortably and offered to show it to him.

"I'm looking at my chest and it's not moving ," he said. "I seem like I'm dead. I'm not seeing any movement of my chest up and down."

I disagreed and pointed to his rhythmic breathing and good chest expansion during the video.

"But this is when I'm really relaxed," he said. "Do you have one from before that?"

I did not; I was intensely caught up in his energy field then.

"I was just curious," he responded. "Right now, I feel pretty good, which is how I feel after all of your sessions. So, it's much better than the way I felt at the beginning."

**"I just went out," he commented. "It's just weird. I was just totally out."**

**Yes, and he was out for a long time, because what he remembered of the session occurred only during the first 30 seconds. After that, for essentially 20 minutes, it seemed Sam's system was working at something.**

**"It was healing," he said. "God, it's like what we were talking about before... Healing usually occurs when you're sleeping. And I was definitely sleeping.**

**"In that dream of getting food onto the plate, it was a sign that something was happening that was trying to work on healing me, just like food is a nutrient. So, the symbolism of the food with something that was essential for me. So, my mind was probably part of the healing process."**

**Sam, however, went back to being haunted by the dream.**

**"The only thing was, every time I would get a little food and pour it on my plate - And it was up rice, because I love rice - Spanish rice, balsamic rice - And I was putting it on there, and I was thinking, 'This is so good.' And all of a sudden, it was like I had a scoop, and what came out was just a very little, few grains. And I'm going, 'I can't... This isn't like a teaspoon of rice.'"**

**"That was my dream," he concluded. "And so maybe my dream was trying to say, 'OK, I'm really close to getting nutrients and maybe healing, but in the long run, I wasn't getting very much..."**

**Our conversation was interrupted when a call came from his doctor's office. Sam provided the details about his Emergency Room visit due to coughing blood, then got off the phone and returned to the subject of our Qi Gong session.**

**He made the comment that he thought that he was active throughout that Qi Gong session, and that's why he was working so hard at breathing throughout the session (even though he was sleeping) until the energy work was done.**

**In other words, when I was actively energetically interacting with him, he was also active; when that energy interaction ceased, he stopped being active, too.**

**So, it suggested mutual effort on both of our parts. And this working together energetically had physical manifestations.**

**"What you were doing was causing me to do something," he asserted. "And since I'm very sensitive of doing something, you could see that with me, whereas you might not see that with other people who are healthier or they will show it in a different way? Mine**

was breathing because I have a lung condition; whereas other people might show it in other ways, based on what their conditions are."

And this even while Sam was sleeping.

"Yes, subconsciously," he affirmed. "It was all in my subconscious. And not in my conscious or awakened state."

And when the energy interaction was over, he wasn't active.

"Yeah, I think any of this stuff can be countered if one really wants to counter it," he said. "But I was not. I mean, you couldn't get more neutral than where I was, because I was sleeping. It was all happening in my subconscious. That's what you were working with… A pure form of my state, versus any state in which there might be resistance or trying to help.

"Because sometimes one tries to help. And it's usually not very productive. You have to let what's really helping you work. You can't aid it. You can't resist it.

"I think sometimes when people try to aid something, they're compensating, and usually most people guess it wrong as to what they're supposed to be doing. So, it's better to let the practitioner do all the controlling when possible.

"I know when Stephen Tamaribuchi is trying to work on my body, and I try to move my body with his movements, then he goes, 'Sam, just let it go. Just let it go. You're interfering with what I'm trying to do.'

"That's a physical thing that he's doing with my joints, and not something at your level. But, still, at your level, I could imagine that things could interfere with it.

"So, from what you're saying about the change in my breathing, that I went from struggling to no struggling… Well, I was totally out of it. I was neutral. I wasn't trying to help you or resist you. The energy from you was 100% working with me in that situation."

"So, the Qi Gong we did today was the most pure form of Qi Gong we've ever done," Sam declared. "Versus when I'm conscious, sitting up. Then, sometimes I'm saying, 'Oh, this feels good', and I'm trying to enhance it more, and sometimes we might not be on the same wavelength?

"I think this is a good way to let you do it, because sometimes my mind is not always correct, and it would be better to just let you take the driver seat.

"It's sort of like having two drivers in one car. Or a backseat driver. He's just trying to help you, but sometimes that help is not very productive."

My Qi Gong mentor, Wah Lee, had expressed doubt about the effectiveness of energetic interactions while the recipient was

**sleeping, saying the recipient had to be able to take things in, and the recipient was capable of that while sleeping. Hence, it was his opinion that you need to be conscious during the energy experience to benefit from it.**

**"In certain circumstances, I'm sure that's the case," Sam affirmed. "But in my situation, I think we made a pretty significant connection and worked even with me out of it - Just relaxed and having me at a buffet table."**

**"But you weren't serving me very well," he added. "You had a hole in the ladle."**

**I held that I was a budding Qi Gong master, not a "dream master", though I did feel the dream needed to be more fully explored.**

**"All the same, it's just interesting," he said. "That's why I say you're exploring new grounds."**

**We certainly had, I responded.**

**I wondered if this was a better way to perform Qi Gong, in general; that is, with people in a supine position on a massage table like this?**

**"I'm glad we were able to do this," he concluded. "From the time we started this the first time until now, you've improved so much. It's pretty good..."**

# CHAPTER SIXTY-FIVE

Monday, June 9, 2025

In a meeting of my "spirit buddies", I shared about my conversation with Sam and trying to address his condition at the primary level; that is, the scarring in his lungs and reversing that by triggering mechanisms of fibrinolysis.

Then, I described Sam's dream, which (for Sam) seemed to cast a shadow on the session.

"So, he did take it in?" Steve asked. "The dream was basically about him saying, 'All of this is in front of me, and I can't take it in. I can't integrate it.' And the dream was about it being a challenge to him. It was a wakeup call. It was an awareness that he needs to open up to be able to take all of this in.

"He sounds like somebody who does so much for other people but doesn't accept stuff for himself. And that's what I think that dream is about. I mean, he puts it all out there for everybody else, but when others put it out there for him, he's unable to take it in. He gets a teaspoon."

April had an additional interpretation.

"My impression was that, at the moment, he can only get a teaspoon of air at a time," she said.

"That was the first thing that I thought," Steve said. "But when Mike went on about the energy, then I had those additional thoughts. But, definitely, there's all that air out there and he's only able to get a teaspoon at a time. And that's sort of a metaphor of his condition. I mean, it's real. It's very, very real. Extremely real. But it's a metaphor for his ability to take as much as he gives.

"And the other thing I was thinking about was Sam saying, 'I can't survive on this.' That's the fear right now. That's the issue: Even though there's so much air out there, he can only take a spoonful at a time, and he's approaching a place where it won't be enough for life."

"But if Mike can help him to heal, that would be amazing," he added, enthusiastically. "I mean, is this something that you have plans to do with him regularly?"

Sam had wondered if this was reproducible and invited me to do this with him again? So, I was planning on going to him right after the three of us spoke.

"That's fantastic," Steve said. "Then you're going today... That would be absolutely amazing. Is there any word at all where he has been placed on the transplant list?"

He still has to do the evaluations to determine if he places at all, I said. That's coming next week.

"Oh, I can't even imagine what that would be like," Steve said. "I know you have to accept life where it is, but that's really hard. That would be so hard…"

Arriving at Sam's, I told him about Sara and Steve's thoughts about his dream.

"I really appreciate that you guys discussed about my dream, and that's really needed, because it does give me more insight," he said. "It's good to get opinions from other people who have much greater knowledge than I do regarding these things. And I want to take it in, as well. It is overwhelming. My mind can only take a little bit at a time. And I do feel starved.

I asked what he thought of Steve's interpretation that Sam gives more than he takes? Sam mostly insisted that he was OK.

"Is the same thing that I tell my relatives," he said. "Just take care of yourself. I'm OK."

"I think what really took me for a tailspin was when my cousin got very, very sick and had to get surgery," he added.

His cousin unfortunately suffered a heart attack while helping to clear Sam's storage.

"And he's just now coming out of it, but he's having difficulties, similar to mine," he continued. "I know he's going to get stronger and better, but he still has to get through this difficult time. For me, it's different, because I'm just going to get worse. I might lose the ability to use my legs, so I won't be able to balance. Every time I take a step, I'll tip over, because I'm just getting weaker. And I'm losing my posture and coordination and that's just one aspect. They'll be other aspects. Like the dryness of my throat. It just keeps getting worse. I won't be able to sleep. It's just all these little things that will continue to degrade my health. Even my talking will start to fade.

"So, I don't think the lack of rice, or lack of food is particular to one particular thing, like breathing. It's with everything else that's happening."

"Anyways, it's just a dream," he declared. "And maybe it's more of a premonition of things to come? A puzzle of a premonition, so that you have to figure out exactly what the meaning is? And overall, you're just going to get a little of everything, and it's just going to get less and less."

"And so, that's my interpretation of it," he concluded. "So, everything steve and sara have said it's right on, except they're trying to be specific…"

He talked about what lay ahead with the lung transplant evaluations.

"I'm treating it as if I climbing Mount Everest," he began. "But here, at least it's a procedure and it's in a controlled environment. Because being on Mount Everest is not a controlled environment. So, you try to prepare for everything. And I've experienced frostbite before.

"Here, at least, I understand that there could be complications, but the variables and chances for those complications don't swing as widely as they do on Mount Everest. So, my chances… Yeah, it's uncomfortable. Yeah, it's a pain in the butt. But you know what? My expedition team is the best. These people know what they're doing. It's not like going up Mount Everest with an unexperienced expedition team. These folks know how to work as a team. They know the rules of survival. My body will be wheeled into an operating room where every person knows exactly what they're supposed to be doing. How amazing is that? All I gotta do is basically live there and let them work on me.

"So, it's not like I'm going up to a razor thin edge on a mountain, inhaling wind, and freezing cold and stinging frost. That's the way I look at it. It's a piece of cake.

"So, I'm looking at it like, 'Yeah, this will be another mountain I can scale.'

"And I think you're helping me. I tell you, whatever you did yesterday, I had that deep sleep and rest. I think that was healing me. I think you kind of directed my body to do something. Because when I woke up this morning, I felt more energetic than I have in the last week or two.

"Because, before that, I could feel myself sinking a little bit more each day. Then, all of a sudden, boom, I got up and I did some exercising, and I did some tai chi, and I felt so good that I did it again!

"And even when I make a mistake when I'm doing tai chi, I'm happy, because I know my body is going to improve on it a little bit more for the next time."

Sam talked about working towards perfecting his Qi Gong technique, then, about his first thoughts when it came to the lung transplant.

"I was thinking, 'Do I want to go through all that? Isn't it better to just exit in a nice way? Make sure I get everything wrapped up? And then slip out the back door?

"But the more I read about the lung transplant and hear stories from people who had it, I go, 'Wow, it is a second chance.'

"However, it is not an easy second chance. But it is a second chance. So, it might be worth it.

"And because of what you did yesterday, I felt like, 'Oh my goodness, I feel better.' And maybe that's what a lung transplant would do? But at a much greater difference."

"But, to get there," he concluded, "I need these little pushes…"

Considering Sam's thoughts about the lung transplant, as difficult as it was, I suppose it was a lot more modest a proposal than what I suggested the day before when I was talking about reversing his condition.

"It's like having the wind at your back when you're hiking," Sam continued. "The wind right now is just a breeze. And I'm hoping that the lung transplant will be gale force winds. So, we'll just take my sails and keep going."

His words made me think about Victor Frankl and what he wrote about in Man's search for meaning about those who survived the Auschwitz concentration camp, saying that those who had expectations that were too high, often got disappointed and those were the ones who ultimately lost hope and perished; whereas those who kept their expectations modest, kept moving forward, and didn't lose hope, were the ones who got through.

"It makes sense," Sam said, "because a little bit of improvement, you feel joy. Versus the people who were expecting big things, so that even when they got a little one, they never felt the joy! Because they were disappointed. Whereas the other people go, 'Oh, man, this is great! I'll take it! Just do a little accomplishment each day, and it all adds up.'

"But it's hard when you're being suppressed. So, I can't blame anyone for giving up. Under that tremendous weight, you lose hope. And it's so easy to lose hope.

"But how does one maintain hope in a disastrous, catastrophic situation?

"But you're right. One such strategy is to enjoy the little things. Let's say it's like a building collapsed on you, and you're trapped. But the ability to at least move your chest so you can take in a breath may be the only joy you have. And if you enjoy it, you go, 'OK, I can make it. Just keep enjoying this ability to move my chest, so that I can at least keep my breath going, and then maybe someone will rescue me.' Versus thinking, 'That little breath is not good enough! I'm going crazy here! I can't move! I'm paralyzed! I wish for death!'"

The latter was how I feared I was.

"That's why I see these people in these situations, and how brave they are, and how strong they are, mentally and physically. These are people who keep the race going. Incredible people.

"And on top of that, they were humane. They helped other people. They kept the other people going, and they were willing to sacrifice themselves for someone else.

"On top of that, they're being crushed. And yet they're trying to help the other person become even better, despite their situation. Incredible people.

"I think that's so important to maintain: Under all that duress is your humanity. That's the thing that always intrigues me. The thing I love about being a human being...

Sam had commented about he needed to get an EKG yesterday, so I couldn't resist showing him the shirt that April got for me that had an EKG against a couple of cat ears.

"That is really cool," Sam said. "There she is – Cat Chow."

I told him the story of how we found Cat Chow (who we first called Socks):

*Taking a walk April turned and stared in the direction of the street.*

*"Oh, that's interesting," she said. "I think we have a stalker."*

*Looking in the direction of her gaze, I saw what appeared as two black triangles that rose just above the curb. A moment later, a kitten lifted and bobbed its head; except for white paws, it was predominantly black.*

*"She looks like she has socks on," April remarked. "I think that's what I'll call her... Socks."*

*April made a clicking sound with her tongue against the roof of her mouth, and the kitten sprang up and came to her, making circles around us.*

*"She wants to come close to me, so I can pet her," she said. "But she's a little scared, because she doesn't know if she can trust me."*

*Then, April's expression changed.*

*"She's been in some fights," she said. "There's a long scar down her ear."*

*Indeed, it appeared as though the kitten's ear had been sliced in two.*

*"Who knows what attacked her," she said.*

*I nodded. It seemed difficult to imagine, seeing how small she was — like a gentle ball of fur.*

*April looked overhead at the darkening sky.*

*"You know there's a storm's coming," she said. "There might be tornadoes, too. I heard over the radio that they were telling everyone who has outdoor pets to bring them inside. I don't know how she's going to make it through all that. You think we could help this kitten through the storm? I know we weren't really planning on having a cat, but maybe we can help this little thing through the storm that's coming."*

*April knelt and held out her hands, but the kitten kept her distance.*

*"It's probably because she doesn't know me very well," she said. "And I don't know her very well, and don't know if she's going to bite me or something."*

*Then, April rose, looking pensive.*

*"I think I'm ready to go home now," she announced.*

*But walking back, April made the clicking sound, and the kitten followed, zipping back and forth in front of us as we made our way.*

*At the house April opened the door; but the kitten remained outside on the stairs, looking in.*

*"She wants to come inside, but she's scared," she said. "And we don't have any cat food. I always heard that if you give them a bowl of milk, they would like that."*

*April put a bowl just inside the door and poured some milk. The kitten sniffed at the milk.*

*"She wants to go in there and get it, but she's still scared," she said. "I can tell she's really hungry and wants it."*

*Then, the kitten got down low and slowly inched forward towards the doorway. She looked outside, and then she looked at the bowl of milk, and then outside again.*

*"She's thinking, 'I want that milk,'" April said.*

*Finally, the kitten crossed the threshold and licked the milk...*

"Yeah, she was the spike," Sam declared. "She was the peak. She was the contraction."

Yes, she became our heartbeat - a part of our hearts. She made her way right into our hearts that day with those two little peak ears against the sidewalk and ever since.

"That is so clever," Sam said. "It's interesting how people come up with these things. I mean, I wonder if the artist was lying in a bed just like I was in the hospital and watching the EKG and saying, 'It's a cat. It's like the ears of a cat.'"

I followed this by telling Sam about the shirt I wore to karaoke that said, "It's weird being the same age as old people." I added, though, that somebody made a slur that night about me being old, referring to me as "Dad."

"You could tell him, 'When you get to my age, you're not going to be able to sing anywhere near as good as I do. You're not going to look anywhere near as good as I do. You're not going to be able to sing as well. Or look as good.'"

"You know, there's a difference there," he asserted. "That's the thing: Getting old is really good if you do it gracefully. That's the trick. In my opinion, If you're gonna be old, you might as well do it gracefully. You don't make yourself look younger; you just fit perfectly into your age. Like you're the poster child of your age. That's what you want to be."

I thought about my father, who was the poster boy for the AARP.

"That's what I always liked about that commercial for Dos Equis - where the Spanish guy, 'Don Juan', who's a really handsome older guy, very sophisticated, and he has his drink, and he's sitting in the leather chair, and even young people would say, 'Oh, I want to be that guy.' It just brought out that age group really well and said, 'If you're this age, you need to look this distinguished'."

And with that, we went and performed Qi Gong…

Performing external Qi Gong with Sam on the massage table again, my right hand entered something of a 'force field' that brought me to Sam's heart chakra, where I first began to experience energy. Again, my hand had to be close before I had that experience of perceiving energy, and again, my hand was stuck like it was in a tractor beam! It would not be moved. I wouldn't move it. There'd have to be a fire in the house before I would move it.

"That's kind of interesting," Sam said. "Because even before you started to say that, I could feel my chest trying to rise up right there in the center of the sternum. Like something was pulling on it."

Again, I couldn't get my hand to move. This was not how I ever experienced energy work. Before it was about following the energy, and if I got out of the path of the energy vector, it was, "Oh, my hand is going out of the path. I need to get my hand back squarely in the energy path again."

This was entirely different, though. This was the energy holding my hand in place. I would not for the life of me pull it out of where it was. There was no element of "self-correcting" here. It was all about the energy determining where it wanted my hand.

It was the same way yesterday, except then it involved my head and especially my upper third eye. Then, my head was stuck in that tractor beam, seemingly sending a pillar of energy towards Sam.

"That's kind of interesting," Sam continued. "My hand, my palms are also feeling energy. Both of them are even in that energy field…"

Minute three

I continued to scan Sam, my hand really low, just a few inches from the surface of his body.

"The energy is leaving my palm now," I said, "but it's moving towards my diaphragm. Like it's trying to pull it down."

I accidentally touched Sam and apologized.

"No, it's interesting," he said. "Because I could feel the energy before you touched me. I was feeling things on my elbow."

That's where I was when I touched him.

"And then it shifted to my diaphragm from my elbows," he said. "It felt like there was something gently pushing on it. Like someone put their thumb and pushed it. It wasn't distinct like the popping feeling, but it felt like a pressure that was pushing on it, very gently on a bubble, but not popping the bubble. Just putting some pressure on it and slightly misshaping it. It felt like it went from the outside of my arm to the inner elbow, more on my right than the left."

I was on his right side.

"But I could feel it on my left, as well," he added. "I can also feel my diaphragm. It's interesting… My thumb feels like it's in a holding pattern. And then my cheeks feel like there's something buzzing there."

It sounded like he was having muscular releases there.

"I don't know what's the deal," he said. "But you never know? They all seem like they're related to my diaphragm for some reason. And if there was a beat, the beat at my cheeks and my arms… They feel like they have a rhythm to it. And it's moving at the same rhythm as the feeling at my diaphragm. Like they're all related. All in sync.

"The difference between yesterday and today is that, yesterday I was mentally fading and falling asleep. I don't feel like falling asleep now. I just feel like I can feel these things at my arms, by the elbow, on the inside of my elbow, my thumbs.

"But there's no feeling at the arms. Just the thumbs. Like the thumbs are kind of locked."

As for me, it felt like I was being directed to move my hand through this energy beachball? And again, this was another new experience for me that I've never had before?

In retrospect, I wonder if this wasn't me moving my hand through Sam's chest wall into his lungs? In a kind of virtual way?

And at the same time, as I was moving my hand through this virtual beach ball energy field, my crown chakra got activated.

"I can feel my forehead and the front of my temple feeling active, too," Sam said. "It's feeling like I can feel different parts of my body like my lower back now. It seems to have come awake or alive?"

My higher third eye became active and held me in place, creating a tractor beam feeling.

Again, before it was always, "OK, I've gone off the path. I have veered off the path. I don't feel the energy as well. It's not as squarely in my hand. I need to get back to the path and follow it the way it's radiating outward." But this has me in a tractor beam! It's holding me. And it's strong.

"There must be a reason for that," Sam said.

The energy put me into a comfortable kneeling position, but still holding my head like it was in a tractor beam and screwed in so that I wouldn't move.

"Yeah, that's not typical," Sam said. "Because usually you're moving all about. Slowly, but you're moving about. This is very odd. Not like something you've ever experienced with me anyway."

It was nothing like I'd ever experienced with anyone...

### Minute 15

"It feels like my body seems to be a little bit free right now," Sam said. "It seems to want to move around. It feels looser. Like my wrist. My fingers. My hands. Before now, I felt all tight.

"Before it was holding my thumbs, and now my thumbs feel relaxed and want to move about."

It felt like there was a beam of energy coming from my upper third eye. And again, I was in a tractor beam.

And it wasn't like a balancing act. I wasn't balancing this energy pillar on top of my head. It wasn't something that was coming down from the heavens to me, and I had to hold myself in place to receive it.

Or maybe it was coming from the heavens, and it was just holding my head there and not giving me a chance to veer off this way or that? I didn't have to hold my head in place just right; instead, it was holding me in place.

'Energy holding you'? I thought, quizzically. 'Tractor beam'?...

Minute 22

Finally, the energy let go of its hold of me, so that I could move about again. I was released from the tractor beam, though I still felt the energy at the top of my head.

"That held you for quite a while," Sam said. "I was really relaxed there, especially at the end."

Sam shifted his gaze.

"You know what?" he said, curious. "I think I'd like to see something."

He retrieved his peak flowmeter and blew into it.

"It's reading 250, which is good," he said.

He then applied his pulse oximeter; the oxygen saturation reading was relatively low at 91%, but his heart rate was 80.

"The heart rate is really good," he said. "Usually my oxygen is higher, so if there is an effect here, there's a slower heart rate and a lower oxygen. I wonder if my body was consuming oxygen more during this time? So maybe even though I was laying down, maybe something was metabolizing more?"

He did seem to be working at something while we were doing this, like his system was active.

"Usually it goes down to 91% when I walk," he said. "But yet my heartbeat was on the lower side."

Yes, heart rate suggested that he was in a relaxed state; oxygen suggested that his system was working at something. Working on something in a relaxed state…

Minute 28

I confided to Sam that I was looking for the long goal of triggering fibrinolysis so for me I was taking a long goal and treating this like running a marathon as opposed to sprint and looking for any instant benefits.

I would, therefore, suggest we take it slow and not expect a lot to happen at once, especially as he was looking to undergo the lung transplant. Hence, all we had to do was help a little bit before he underwent that procedure.

"Yes, that's my goal," Sam said. "Getting through the lung transplant in a better way. That's what I'm hoping for. So, I have to keep working at that. But this seems to be making me feel good. Like right now I feel less stressed and like my body is functioning better. If I was to guess, I would've expected the peak flow to be higher. And 250 - I'll take that. Because sometimes I get down to 200…"

I reiterated my surprise at feeling energy as though I was in a tractor beam.

"So, you're experiencing new stuff," he said. "Because it seems like you did a lot more walking around before when you were first doing it with me. I used to remember, thinking, 'Wow, Mike is way out there. And now here you are feeling like you are locked, which is really interesting. Do you get that with other people?"

No, this was the first time I had ever had this kind of experience.

"Wow, that's really interesting," Sam responded. "That 'locking up'? I wonder if it will show a significant healing that's occurring and if things start to improve? As I've said, I'm just looking for tiny improvements…"

Sam asked if I'd been interacting with folks from Yale University itself? I said, again, that Ellen had reached out to some of the university folks on my behalf to consider the question of a spiritual component in my Qi Gong efforts?

"'Spiritual'," Sam repeated. "What does it actually mean? Same question goes for religion. What really is religion? Is religion 100% man-made to control other people? Religion has a big umbrella. It covers so much. It has so many spokes to it. That's why it's such a big enterprise - 'We have something for everyone. Even if you're agnostic. There's a spoke for you'…"

Sam indicated that he didn't want to keep me late; however, as he was escorting me outside, he commented that it wasn't just me feeling like I was in a tractor beam.

**"It was me, too," he said. "I was feeling it at my thumbs. They didn't want to move. They were just stuck in one place..."**

# CHAPTER SIXTY-SIX

Tuesday, June 10, 2025.

After the "tractor beam" experience with Sam, I had a night of intense dreaming.

I wondered that what was going on that, having been connected with what felt like Sam's entire nervous system, if there wasn't some energetic passing of the entirety of Sam's experience and wisdom onto me? That's probably the reason that I'm having all of these realizations, I thought. That's why things are finally coming together after all this time. For example, the resolutions of feelings about Bubbles - this forty-years after our relationship.

He is right, I concluded. I need this more than he does.

However, as well as the night of intense dreaming, I was also experiencing chest tightness and reached out to my Hakomi therapist, Jackie.

Hakomi Therapy amounts to body-centered psychotherapy. Today, I talked with Jackie about my childhood traumas, like being struck in the chest by my uncle, feeling unsupported by my parents, and wondering if my symptoms were related to a need to hold my chest tight, so to "protect my heart."

Jackie probed by asking the question, "Notice in your body if anything changes when you hear me say, 'Mike, you can let all of that go.'"

Energy became activated at my upper third eye, to which I reacted with my objective mind by thinking, "No, duh. Of course, there's a conflict between higher ideals (like letting go) and survival tendencies; however, along with this, I experienced worsening chest tightness. So, there was this "cognitive dissonance": On the one hand, the response was like, "Of course"; on the other, the emotional response seemed to be, "No, you can't do that. I have to protect my heart from that." Hence, emotionally, it seemed to me that I didn't want to let go. I was afraid of letting go.

"The things I'm wondering about is whether there are things in your relationship with Sam that are keeping it from changing?" Jackie said. "And change is going to happen one way or the other. Because things change, and neither you nor Sam nor I nor anybody is able to change that."

She commented about the mantra held by a colleague.

"He says, 'You let go of anything between you and inner peace.' So, you're just letting go of everything that stands between you and inner peace. It's kind of like a clearing."

Yeah, but if Sam were to let go of anything that was getting in the way of inner peace, he'd be letting go of life, because his body is getting in the way of inner peace, I thought. His lungs are getting in the way of inner peace. And to let go of that, was to let go of life, it seemed to me. The thing between him and inner peace was getting enough air. If he were to let go of getting enough air, he'd be dead.

"Energy doesn't dissipate," Jackie shared in conclusion. "It transforms. It doesn't cease to exist. Transformation occurs. That's why energy medicine works. We just don't understand all of the energy…"

After the Hakomi Therapy session, I went to Sam's again to perform Qi Gong. Talking beforehand, Sam said that he felt his health was slipping, but felt the Qi Gong was having a positive effect.

"I'm going to tell you," he began, "not just this, but also the internal Qi Gong sessions on the teleconference. That felt positive. I think that's because you and the two other people were really into it, so they were more positive, and I think maybe that vibe was strong, too - The group interaction. Because I felt really comfortable with both of them. I kind of wonder if there were more if I wouldn't have an even better feeling? Like an even more combined effect?

Yes, the members of my Qi Gong group had a firm belief that the more members involved, the more powerful the experience, though I didn't think that was anything that had passed the rigors of clinical study.

"No," Sam said. "No, but I'm feeling stronger. In fact, I'm improving. As a matter of fact, let me show you my red book where I keep my notes."

He pulled out the book from the top of the side table next to his chair in the living room and review it with me.

"Today, I blew at 280," he indicated. "But before I was hovering at 240, 220, 210. But then, after the treatment, it went up to 280. And what's really interesting is, I didn't think I blew that hard and yet it was the highest. I just blew into it and the thing shot up higher than it ever did. So, maybe what we're doing is really helping?..."

He said his Shiatsu therapist, Stephen Tamaribuchi, was coming to his home to work with him.

"He's going to work physically on my body, which will be really great, because my hip is hurting, and also my knee, so I don't want to move around as much," Sam said. "So, I figure if I could keep things in my body going, then it will help.

"One thing is, I noticed that I'm not coughing as much. But my what I call 'hiccupping' during exhalation is still there, and I'm hoping that that will decrease, as well."

Yes, that was probably what was responsible for sending fluid into his airways that led to that choking episode, in which he coughed blood. It's probably also what's putting him at risk of asphyxiation pneumonia.

"So, I think I'm optimizing my situation," he continued. "And it's depressing without that, because it's hard. It's difficult if I want to do things."

He asked about my day? I told him that I'd requested sick leave today because I'd a moment of weakness and wanted to talk with my therapist.

"You didn't go to work today?" he responded. "Now, I'm worried about you."

I immediately regretted having told him and insisted there were just these issues that were surfacing in me.

"Even if it has nothing to do with me, there's something happening with you," he correctly deduced.

I told him a half-truth, saying that I got a call from Bubbles, and it led to the surfacing of some deep-seated emotions.

"She reached out to you?" he asked. "You didn't reach out to her?"

As a matter of fact, it was because I had told her about what was going on with him that she reached out to me, saying that she felt like she knew Sam from my letters and how important he was to me, so she was concerned.

Indeed, I'd invited her to join the Qi Gong group virtually, because it was an experience with Bubbles that led to the development of the Qi Gong self-practice.

"I didn't know that," Sam responded. "But it makes sense."

I told him about that experience. It started when her mother had a heart attack while visiting her in Las Vegas. At the time, pebbles told me that the only thing that the doctor said would help her mother was a heart transplant, which then got me thinking about Sam, being that doctors were now saying that the only thing that would help him was a lung transplant!

But Bubbles had gone on that her mother was too weak for the procedure because she had developed an ulcer and wasn't eating (Again, there were similarities to Sam).

So, where there was nothing else to help her mother, I volunteered to go out and help with bioenergy.

Ultimately, her mother was able to eat, got her strength back, they performed a cardiac procedure, which turned out to be a corner artery bypass so to attempt to get her heart beyond the stunned myocardium state from a heart attack, and the procedure went well.

And finally, when I left them, I expected to experience that sense of sadness that happened every time I left them. But instead of sadness for remorse, it felt like I was within this cocoon of energy that I felt on that bus ride home.

Thirty years later, when I'm assigned the scientific mentor at the VA, the mentor tells me that the reason she took me on was because a friend did work like I did, and he wanted to meet me, and asked me to talk with him.

When I reached out to the friend, he said that he wanted me to work with him virtually. I had never done that before, and tried to somehow reach out and connect with him energetically by transposing his energetic circulation on mine, and looking for energy disturbances that way.

And then I had an experience with him like the one that I had on that bus ride.

Long story, short, those sessions lead to the development of my Qi Gong self-practice.

"Makes sense," Sam said. "It's nice to hear about its progression…"

Performing external Qi Gong with Sam, I immediately encountered something I'd never experienced before: There was this really narrow line of energy that was taking me down his midline and activating my crown chakra. And the energy path was so thin and light and wanted to interact mostly with the back of my ring finger. And I felt something of an energy ring around my wrist, too.

I was following the energy with my right hand, but my left hand was also activated and felt energy just at my ring finger there, too.

"You think it's saying that this process involves all kinds of parts of your body?" Sam asked. "Because I think if you're just expecting something to just happen at the palm of your hand, you're limiting your possibilities. I think you need to just let it flow wherever it leads. Because there are other connections there that are vital and need to be more optimized to work."

He described how it was that for headaches there was a prescribed acupuncture point between the thumb and the index finger that you were supposed to rub to get relief.

"Go figure?" he said. "Why does the web of your hand have an effect on your headache? That's kind of a mystery, but yet there is a connection between your head and that web.

"So, basically when you're doing this thing, you never know what part of your body has a connection with the point where I need help on my body?"

It was just a matter of following the energy for me, I responded. Perhaps there was something in traditional Chinese medicine teachings that could explain all of this, and there was a connection between this thin line of energy at his midline and the ring finger, but I was aware of it.

"Yeah, so maybe just asking somebody who is a Qi Gong master and see if they match it with what you're experiencing," he suggested.

I stayed quiet, though internally I was feeling frustrated and recalling the words of one of the Long COVID-Qi Gong participants (M.), who would respond to such questions by saying, "Show me the double-blind!"

In other words, it's not scientific; it's all observational. There's not a Qi meter to measure and study and quantitate and really analyze or be able to offer anything with some semblance of intelligible thing to say about any of this. Let's just hope there is something to this and it helps.

Sam wanted to know more about the thin line of energy I was perceiving.

"Is it near my belly?" he asked.

I had begun to perceive it at his chest, but, currently, yes, I was at his belly, just under the navel.

"I can feel that," he said. "I feel something right around here."

His eyes closed, he exactly indicated where my hand was above his body.

"And that's weird," he added, "because I had my eyes closed all the time, and I could feel my stomach being pulled up a bit."

Yes, another member of the post study group (W.) had described such an experience that seemed to involve the "Sushumna", which, according to Ayurvedic Medicine, is the central energetic line that flows from the top of the head to the base of the spine and supports the flow of Prada/Qi.

On one occasion, while working with W., she said that she felt like what sounded like her sushumna being pulled outwards and towards me in a forward direction. At the time I had been perceiving energy over her midline chakras, and, even more interesting, I was facing her, which is unusual because I typically avoid this and stand to the side of recipients, so not to assume a posture that was suggestive of being aggressive, forceful or overly assertive while performing external Qi Gong.

In "Practice Energy Healing in Integrity; the Joy of Offering Your Gifts Legally & Ethically", Midge Murphy states, "In Eastern Indian traditions, the sushumna is the central energetic line that flows from the top of the head to the base of the spine and supports the flow of the basic life force or Prada. When we are in harmony with the central core of our being, imaged as this straight energetic line, we are at one with ourselves and the world around us. However, a single event, word, gesture, or negative intention can throw us off, putting us out of balance..."

"There is a connection between my chest and my stomach," Sam continued. "Because I tell you, my appetite is just weirded out, and that it feels like my stomach is hollow, but it doesn't want to accept anything. But today it was so much better. I ate things and it felt good and it wasn't bothering me."

Sam continued that the point was just above his belly button and wondered if the sushumna could be related to the parasympathetic?

"Do you think it has anything to do with the vagus nerve?" he asked.

According to Ayurvedic Medicine, the Sushumna didn't skew towards favoring the parasympathetic nervous system, but, rather, represented a neutral space of balance between the sympathetic and parasympathetic; it was, however, associated with Kundalini awakening, described as a transformative spiritual process where dormant, coiled energy—symbolized as a serpent at the base of the spine—rises through the chakras to the crown, resulting in expanded consciousness.

*Often called "Shakti" or divine feminine energy, this "coiled snake" represents dormant spiritual potential, and its awakening is*

***associated with intense, sometimes physically palpable, spiritual and energetic shifts…***

Minute 21

More than just my ring finger, I was feeling energy at my thumb, as well as the activation of energy around my navel or Dantian. My hands were rhythmically moving in and out now, as though following the breathing of some energy ball.

Next, my hands stopped, and there was this feeling of energy around my loins. Then, the energy left my hands, so that it was mostly in my head and directed me downwards into a squat, which I assumed with such ease that it surprised me - like it required no effort at all, and I didn't feel it in my quads.

"What do you think is the reason for squatting or getting down so low?" Sam asked.

I thought that it might be that it was because all of this energy coming out of my head could be sent in his direction, as it felt like it was coming out of my head like some ring of Saturn.

"Laterally," Sam said.

Yes, and with me in the squatting position, it just seemed like it was better able to be directed at him. That was my guess. Especially as the squatting position was different, as I usually do things like kneel when the energy directs me downwards.

Finally, the energy directed me to sit cross legged on the floor, the energy from my head still coming out of me laterally towards Sam.

My eyes were closed, and I was seeing this fluid yellow moving about and tumbling around and very pleasant to watch.

"It sounds like a lava lamp," Sam correctly deduced.

I commented that I'd never been on LSD, but I imagine this was what it would be like to be on a very pleasant "trip".

Still sitting with this pleasant energy at the top of my head, I wasn't having that tractor beam experience, though I wasn't in a position to want to be moving my head any different way, so I couldn't be sure.

"Maybe you're progressing?" Sam said.

Whatever it might be, I hoped it was giving Sam what he needed.

I reminded him about his comments of finding the things were most significant the first time you did them, and then, afterwards, they become less so.

"I just thought doing this in the series, you could see a progression," Sam said. "It's sort of like moving a big rock or big boulder, I should say; and if you stop and mess around, the boulder goes back; but by continuing to push it, you get it to move forward, rather than it moving back. Because if you give it too much time, it will move back.

"And I was thinking that this would be a good opportunity for you to study your external chi going a little bit more, because I'm pretty much the perfect subject for you, being this far along in my illness and with a greater sensitivity."

To say nothing of what he meant to me…

Minute 32

I felt an impulse to open my eyes, so signal the end of the session.

"That was pretty powerful," Sam said. "Because my stomach feels much better. I appreciate that, Mike."

"So, when will you be seeing Bubbles?" he asked.

She said she wanted me to visit with her on July 5th.

He expressed surprise.

"I thought she was back east?" he said. "In Tennessee?"

No, I said Tennessee was where I followed Kate and the kids. Bubbles lived in Las Vegas.

"I didn't know she was so close," he responded. "It's funny that you didn't see her sooner?"

I shared that we'd actually got together last year in Fairfield.

"So, you have been in contact with her," he said. "That is wonderful."

I said that being away from her by going to the East Coast was among one of the most troubling things to me when it came to going to yale. Just a thought of being on the other side of the continent and that far away from her, with that much distance between us.

"Yeah, but I think your development in this field of Qi Gong is very important," he responded. "And it could benefit Bubbles in the future. Just as you had helped her mom."

I shared with Sam how it was that when I told Bubbles that there was this issue that the position could be taken away because of what was going on with the government, she lamented that, saying she felt what I was doing had a lot to give to humankind.

"Exactly," Sam said. "So that's why it's important to pursue it and not worry about whether it's going to be defunded or whatever.

You'll find a way to keep pushing forward. Unless there's a crisis in your life, so that you have to pull back.

"I mean, if I was worried about what was going to happen to me earlier in my life, I would never have done anything. And I wouldn't have achieved things that made me happy and feel like I have no regrets.

"So, if you worry about things that haven't happened, and you don't know that they will happen, that even though you're trying to be so cautious, you've got to look at if what you're going to gain anything more with chi gong outweighs something that would detour your path?

"Because, yeah, you'll be detoured for a while, but you'll find another path. And then you're farther ahead of the road."

I knew he was completely right, and my feelings were without reason or logic, and spoke to problems I have… Something unfulfilled in childhood that makes this person so important to me.

"Right," he said. "But she's not going to go away. And you can always fly back.

"I don't know. I believe what really makes you happy is this Qi Gong. I think you told me that so many times.

"And for you to not pursue it, I think you would regret it in the end.

"If yale continues its program and it got funded and you decided not to go there, I think that would hurt you more. I mean, if you don't go, you would be more about wanting to destroy the program. So that you'd be saying, 'Gee, I hope it really dissolves…. Because I'm not there… And it justifies my reasoning for not going there. So, I hope an atomic bomb or something drops on their program.'"

Yes, because I'd be filled with regret.

"Yeah," he said, compassionately, "and I don't think you want that to happen. You'd rather say, 'If it's going to happen there and it does dissolve, I want to be on ground zero, and I'm going to survive that ground zero. I'll be one of the survivors because I have this will to survive…"

Minute 41

I told Sam that I'd miss working with him and it was one of the reasons I was conflicted about going off to Yale.

"I think you'll keep pursuing what you're doing here when you're at yale to a certain extent," he responded. "And then you'll be able to write about this experience with an even stronger focus when you're over there in the program. Because you're going to be

**gathering more information and putting the pieces together, so that you're going to be putting the puzzle together.**

**"That's what I think. But you need to satisfy your basic needs of finance and making sure you don't lose what you've already gained. Maybe you work at the VA hospital part time over there? And with your experience and résumé, they'll go, 'Yeah, we need you on our staff.' And so, you'll be getting income on top of the fellowship. I would work out those types of details. It's sort of a burden on you, but at least you'll be doing the two things that make you happy.**

**"Because if you stayed here - Which I would love you to stay, because, my goodness, you've been such a great friend and an aid to me - But I think you need to be over there, gathering more information. So that when I do see you again, you'll be really able to help me! Because you'll be so much more powerful in your ability to understand this form of practice.**

**"And I see it already, because I believe you're so much better today than you were when you first started working with me. Maybe it's because I'm more sensitive to it? I can't discard that. But if I try to remove that variable, I think that you're just more focused. You're more capable of getting to the heart of my issues sooner and quicker.**

**"And my link with you is stronger, too. Because now I can have my eyes closed, and I can pretty much know where your hands are. Because I didn't open my eyes, and my stomach was feeling it, and your hand was over my stomach. And I figured, 'Yeah, it must be that his hand is above my stomach, because my stomach is where I'm feeling it.'"**

**"So, you're establishing a link with your patients," he concluded…**

**Before leaving, Sam and I talked about polyvagal theory, in particular as it related to retained energy of trauma and the freeze response and whether when you release retained energy of trauma from a freeze response, what you're doing is removing the stimulation from the dorsal vagal parasympathetic and getting folks back to the Ventral vagal state?**

**"What interests me," he declared, "is why would one branch contain such a severe reaction?"**

**Because you need it, I responded.**

**I explained to Sam the ventral vagal freeze response as described by Peter Levine; namely, when the gazelle is being chased by the cheetah, and the cheetah is about to pounce, the dorsal vagal is triggered because it's the gazelle's only chance and last escape mechanism. All hope on the cheetah having been chasing the gazelle**

out of instinct rather hunger, which happens one time out of 10. Hence, you have a 10% chance of survival if you activate the freeze response.

"It's your last Hail Mary," Sam correctly stated. "Too bad it doesn't work with headlights coming at you. Out in the wilderness there's no predator out there with high beams."

"I'm wondering why some people remain pretty cool under duress, and other people freeze up?" he continued. "Like I'm under duress a lot, but people think I'm still functioning fine until I choke. And when I choke, my breathing just freezes, and I have to really try hard to get it going again."

"I can imagine that that dorsal branch got activated when I got the water stuck there," he said of his recent choking episode. "I couldn't breathe. I just froze. And I had to force myself, and that's why I probably ruptured my throat and bled trying to get my breathing to kick in."

"Because it's scary when I get to that point when I just freeze," he continued. "I think I developed that because when I was drowning, I froze... I froze my breathing, so that I wouldn't get the water into my lungs - The salt water.

"And, so, I remember that last moment. And ever since then, my breathing has been difficult in the sense of the timing. And maybe that's why I couldn't do Tai Chi very well for the longest time? Because I couldn't get my breathing right with my movements. In a lot of movements in Tai Chi, you're supposed to breathe in, and then you release it and exhale. That was really difficult for me. I would always get it mixed up - But only after my drowning."

"Because it threw me totally off," Sam declared. "Trying to lock up my airway.

"So, thinking about this, I think I learned to activate that dorsal branch sooner. So, after the drowning, I noticed that I would get more into a paranoid situation where I always thought, 'Gee, when I get into danger, I use 'cool, calm and collected' to figure it out.' I figure I was just playing with a ventral branch, so I was able to stay in that ventral branch and never jump into that dorsal branch."

"But now, I can jump into that dorsal branch very easily," he concluded, "and that scares me…"

I suggested that perhaps the reason why he had the difficulty with his breathing while performing tai chi was because of residual retained energy of trauma at the dorsal branch? And perhaps we could release that retained energy of trauma, so to get his system working more optimally?

Sam countered that he thought he'd delt with that problem.

"After many years and due to this illness," he began, "I've been forcing myself to learn to try to breathe with my stomach and get the Tai Chi timing down.

"And so, I've been working on that. I work on it at night. I fall asleep working on it. And that's why I think that Tai Chi has begun to come easier for me.

"Because I think there's three things: There's the breathing. There's the leg movements. There's the upper body movements. And the fourth thing is the synchronization. And I see that once I go into the dorsal vagal, I lose all synchronization. And it just wants me to freeze. And if I freeze, I can't breathe."

I nodded, though, at the same time, I wondered: Both Sam and I had experienced the activation of the dorsal branch of the vagus nerve; it came at a time when both of us were drowning (me caught in an undertow, and Sam pulled out to sea). Its activation probably saved my life and made it so I entered a suspended state of animation until I was pulled out of the undertow by that lifeguard.

But nobody pulled Sam out – he just hit the bottom of the ocean floor, and then, it struck him he could probably fight a little further to get to shore; so, he pulled himself out of that dorsal vagal state and put himself into sympathetic again. So, it makes sense that his system was significantly more traumatized and he'd have more retained energy of trauma there.

And it was beautiful to be in that dorsal vagal state; as well as putting me in a suspended state of animation, it also flooded by system with endorphins, so to create a state of tranquility and peace like I never knew (before or since!).

But what of my friend? Would it work for him that way when he needed it now? Or was he right to be worried, and his system was wrecked this way, and there was so much retained energy of trauma there from his previous near-drowning episode that it wouldn't give him relief when he called on it; but, rather, put him in a frozen state in which he couldn't breathe and intensify his horror?...

# ABOUT THE AUTHOR

Michael Yanuck MD PhD is a physician-scientist whose groundbreaking research at the National Institutes of Health was the basis for an FDA-approved vaccine for cancer. Following a traumatic leg injury, he trained in Bioenergy and Qi Gong, introduced Energy Medicine techniques at the National Center for Complementary and Integrative Health, and worked with Chi Gong Masters who were part of the President's Executive Committee on Alternative Medicine. For his work with Veterans in the VA Innovation Accelerator-Qi Gong project, he received the 2023 Science of Tai Chi & Qigong Award from Harvard University and co-led the University of California-Davis Long COVID-Qi Gong project, providing hope to those with long COVID.

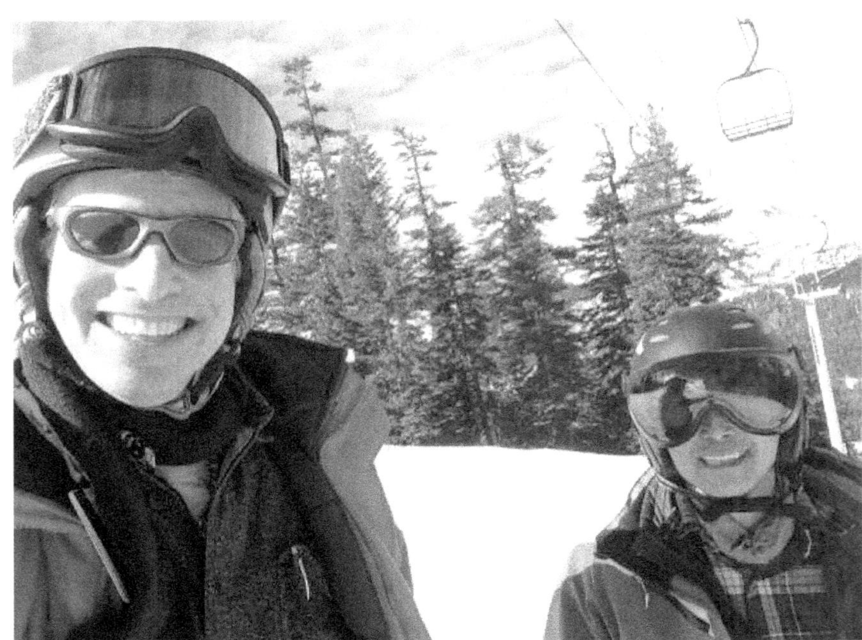

www.ingramcontent.com/pod-product-compliance
Lightning Source LLC
LaVergne TN
LVHW020044110826
845155LV00029B/630

* 9 7 8 1 9 4 6 6 0 0 4 7 9 *